Y0-ACH-770

TRANSLATED FROM THE ORIGINAL FRENCH AND
FIRST PUBLISHED IN AN ENGLISH EDITION
WITH THE AID OF A GRANT MADE
TO YALE UNIVERSITY BY
THE JANE COFFIN CHILDS MEMORIAL FUND
FOR MEDICAL RESEARCH

THE RIDDLE OF CANCER

BY

CHARLES OBERLING M.D.

TRANSLATED BY WILLIAM H. WOGLOM M.D.

NEW HAVEN
YALE UNIVERSITY PRESS
LONDON · HUMPHREY MILFORD · OXFORD UNIVERSITY PRESS
1944

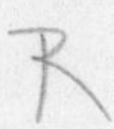

Printed in the United States of America

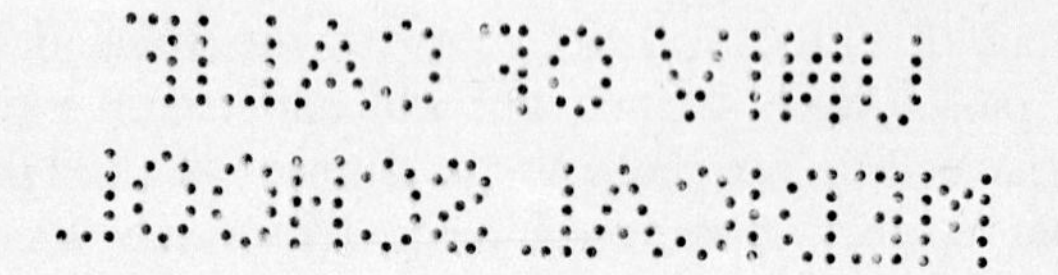

AUTHOR'S PREFACE

THIS book was born of a series of lectures given by the author before the Cancer Institute of the Faculty of Medicine of Paris and the Faculty of Medicine of Teheran. Thus it is addressed particularly to medical students and to those physicians desirous of some acquaintance with the trend of cancer research today. But because of the widespread interest in the cancer problem it seemed worth while to make the book accessible to a still larger public by omitting, wherever possible, any discussion of details and by explaining such technical terms as must of necessity be employed.

Obviously this book is not for the specialist, that is to say, the oncologist. Even the briefest account of our knowledge would fill many volumes, nor could it be undertaken by one person alone. The domain is so broad and invades so many branches of science that to treat the subject adequately an author would have to be at once physicist, chemist, geneticist, bacteriologist, pathologist, parasitologist, and, last but not least, internist, surgeon, and radiologist. All that can be offered in a book like this are general ideas, sketches of a whole field, and brief summaries of experimental investigations. There can be no question of completeness, of citing every relevant article, or of developing each point in accordance with its merits.

The student of cancer will not reproach me, then, if he finds some of his work passed by in silence, but will understand that I have been limited by space and even more by the purpose of the book.

In another respect, however, I have deliberately incurred the displeasure of many colleagues, and that is by defending the virus hypothesis.

In justification I can say that my view is not a preconceived idea, neither was it a part of my medical background. Masson, a prominent cytologist who guided my first steps in the study of cancer, naturally preferred a cellular explanation, Boveri's theory in particular. On the other hand Roussy, with whom I had the honor of working for more than ten years, had an abiding horror of partisanship in scientific matters, and so keen was his desire to recognize the kernel of truth in every conjecture that he was inevitably led to accept a multiple etiology, and to seek the ultimate cause in mutation. Borrel, of a temperament exactly opposite, defended his ideas passionately against all and despite all—sometimes even against the evidence. So at least it seemed with cancer, for I was one of a group that listened to his arguments, admiring his seductive eloquence and fertile imagination, swept away by his enthusiasm, but believing not a single word in his tales of viruses that are ubiquitous and able to work their way along from cell to cell until, at some auspicious moment, they encounter a susceptible one and end by initiating the malignant change.

If the words of Borrel awoke but few echoes it was because they were uttered at a time when it required the greatest courage to maintain the virus hypothesis. Furthermore, he was consistently delayed in completing the proof of his discoveries, parasitic sarcoma of the rat among others, by his extraordinary confidence in his own judgment, which would admit no doubt, and by his almost uncanny perception of weak points in the arguments and experiments of others. Yet Borrel made predictions that should have struck, as they did me, all those who were privileged to discuss with him the problems of cancer. He foresaw that there would be failures at times in attempts to produce malignant growths with Spiroptera, insisted that parasites take part in the spreading of viruses, and suspected from the first that in the so-called hereditary cancer of mice something other than genetic factors may be transmitted. More than once I have heard him suggest the passage of some agent by way of the milk.

All these predictions have been realized, and one cannot help being impressed thereby, particularly since it has now been shown that viruses are instrumental in eliciting a whole series of tumors, benign and malignant. I often think that the wide distribution of the viruses and their important role in disease remain totally unrealized. Indeed, their presence and multiplication within the cell and their selective action on certain parts of it make them today the only plausible explanation of the malignant change, even though the intervention of other factors is recognized.

But as this is a logical postulate rather than a demonstration, I intend to indicate in the closing chapter, in order that the reader may not be misled, the dividing line between fact and theory. A hypothesis is valuable only in so far as it does not flagrantly controvert the known facts, and the virus hypothesis satisfies the requirement. Tomorrow, however, this may not be the case, for in spite of our troubled times science develops so rapidly that any day may contribute new and wholly unexpected information. Yet even though our conceptions should have to be revised almost overnight we shall be easily consoled, for our aim is not the confirmation of an idea but the solution of a problem. Unfortunately all are likely to go astray in that quest for, as Fontana wrote, in 1781, research is a game of chance in which the probability of error is great and that of discovering the truth small.

C. O.

Mary Imogene Bassett Hospital,
Cooperstown, New York.

TRANSLATOR'S PREFACE

THE author of this book is a prominent figure among European students of cancer. Author, teacher, investigator, he has explored every part of the field until there can be but little with which he is not thoroughly familiar. He speaks, therefore, with authority, and the general reader may be congratulated that he has now turned his great talents to the production of a popular treatise on the cancer problem.

For the benefit of this reader it should be explained that, like all who specialize in cancer research, Professor Oberling uses the word *cancer* indiscriminately for any malignant tumor, whereas the surgeon and the general pathologist restrict it to epithelial tumors, employing *sarcoma* for those that spring from connective tissue. This, no doubt, because the experimentalist is interested solely in the nature of the malignant process, which appears to him to be identical no matter what the origin of the growth.

Perhaps it should be explained, also, that *tumor* is an all-inclusive term, like *neoplasm,* or *new growth,* applied to any group of independently growing cells whether they be malignant or benign. Thus all cancers are tumors but, fortunately, all tumors are not cancers.

Translation has been called pouring from a golden into a silver goblet. The translator earnestly hopes that his will prove to be of no baser metal.

W. H. W.

New York,
October, 1943.

CONTENTS

Author's Preface v

Translator's Preface vii

I. Why Should Cancer Interest Us? 1

II. Development of Knowledge on the Nature of Cancer 10

III. Three Hypotheses 17
The Irritation Hypothesis 18
The Embryonal Hypothesis 26
The Microbic or Parasitic Hypothesis 33

IV. Experimental Cancer 38
The Transplantable Tumor 40
Conditions Essential to Success 40
The Behavior of Transplanted Cancer 44
Changes in the Structure of Transplanted Tumors and the Appearance of New Tumors 50
Influence of Various Factors on the Development of a Graft and the Problem of Immunity 51
The Induced Tumor 59
Carcinogenic Rays 59
Parasites as a Cause of Cancer 66
Hereditary Factors in Cancer 75
Carcinogenic Chemical Compounds 87
The Tar Tumor 89
The Carcinogenic Hydrocarbons 94
The Carcinogenic Viruses 110
General Nature of the Viruses 111
Virus Tumors 129

V. Conclusion: One Kind of Cancer or Many? 150
Viruses and Neoplasms Ascribed to Parasites 157
Viruses and Tumors Ascribed to Chemical Agents 159
Viruses and Tumors Ascribed to Heredity 160

Bibliography 170

Index 189

THE RIDDLE OF CANCER

I

WHY SHOULD CANCER INTEREST US?

"CANCER is the failure of medicine." This accusation, so often heard, reflects the bitterness of public opinion in the face of a defeat to which it must be peculiarly sensitive, since medicine has many other humiliating failures to its account.

Speak of someone who has heart disease, or tuberculosis, and you will hear only the conventional manifestations of pity or of sympathy, but let the conversation turn to a patient with cancer and you will see an expression suddenly frozen in horror. Questioning begins forthwith, to end invariably with that pathetic exclamation: When will they ever find a cure for this terrible scourge?

Cancer makes a vivid impression upon almost everyone as physicians well know, for they are harassed by persons otherwise entirely rational who live in constant dread of this disease. These "cancerophobes" end by becoming nervous wrecks. Every little pain, every loss of weight, every slight ailment real or imaginary, is interpreted as a sure sign, whipping fear into a paroxysm of terror and making life unendurable for these unfortunates and for their families as well.

Nothing illustrates better the wide extent of this obsession than the welcome given to patent medicines that are supposed to ward off the malady. It is practically certain that not one of these products has ever prevented a single cancer from developing, yet the unscrupulous dealers who prescribe them reap an astonishing harvest.

Why this fear of cancer? The question is complex, for many facts combine to make the disease a symbol of terror.

In the first place, its name has a mysterious and disquieting sound, and no one has ever really understood why Hippocrates chose it. Was it to portray the outline of certain cancers of the breast, whose ramifications suggest a crab with its claws buried in the living flesh? Or was it to describe the gnawing, shooting pain caused by those claws? Nobody knows. But the name, perhaps on account of its enigmatic quality, brings to mind with singular clarity the condition to which it belongs.

Again, the nature of the malady inspires fear. The stealthy attack, slow yet irrevocable; the depression, so different from the buoyancy of tuberculosis; the ulceration, with its fetid secretion; the loss of flesh, giving the advanced cancer patient, with his emaciated, cadaverous face, the aspect of one dead and forgotten among the living: all these stamp on the memory of those who have watched such a person die an ineffaceable impression of suffering and horror.

It would be wrong, however, to think that this train of events is always present. The prevailing impression is much worse than the reality, for often the suffering is no more severe than in other disorders. It should be realized that cancer in itself is not painful and that it may exist for a long time without causing the least trouble. Indeed, it is precisely this that gives the disease its insidious character, a feature that frequently delays its diagnosis and hence the timely institution of appropriate treatment.

Another factor that has contributed to the fear of cancer is the widely prevalent belief that it is hereditary. Many a woman passes her life in terror because her mother died of cancer of the breast or uterus, and many a man because his father's or grandfather's death was brought about by cancer of the stomach. "Cancer is in the family" they say, and feel themselves the victims of an inexorable fate from which no human hand can rescue them.

We shall see later that the heredity of cancer is a problem far from simple. Nevertheless, the general public believe that the malady is inherited, and it is hard to rid their minds of an idea that has for them all the semblance of truth.

Thus the fear of cancer is a reality to be reckoned with, but this in itself does not explain the interest aroused by the disease. There are other afflictions at least as terrible and others again that are just as inevitably fatal. So if cancer has become one of the great problems of the day, enlisting the interest of experimentalists, sociologists, and even of governments, it must be for reasons more objective, more serious, than simple fear, no matter how widespread this may be.

Now the social importance of a disease, apart from its gravity, depends largely on its frequency. But whoever attempts to investigate cancer from this point of view immediately runs into serious difficulties. All that is known of its frequency has been gathered from vital statistics, which, so far as causes of death are concerned, are based upon death certificates furnished by physicians or government officials. Unfortunately these statements are so little subject to supervision that almost anything may be set down thereon, and in the case of cancer their unreliability is multiplied still further by false entries, made in deference to the wishes of relatives who do not want the word cancer to appear on the record.

Even though these documents are filled out conscientiously they may still be vitiated by numerous errors. Many cancers can be diagnosed in the living patient only by procedures that are not available to the country doctor, and even in the perfectly equipped hospitals of great cities some escape the most accurate clinical examination and are not found until autopsy. Thus only statistics that are founded upon autopsy findings can reflect the real frequency of cancer, and such statistics do not exist. Even in those countries where post-mortem examination is widely practiced, hardly 10 per cent of the dead come to autopsy.

So the reliability of statistics on the frequency of cancer depends in great measure on the prevailing conditions of sanitary equipment and organization, the care with which the disease is sought out, and the accuracy of death certificates. If cancer seems to be commoner in cities than in rural districts this is only because it is more often recognized on account of the larger number of doctors and the better facilities for examination. It is the same, too, with differences in frequency among the various countries. If the recorded mortality from cancer per 100,000 inhabitants is 140 in Denmark, 124 in Switzerland, 116 in England, 105 in Germany, 100 in Holland, 84 in France, and 50 in Spain and Italy, this means simply that the highest numbers come nearer the truth.

The real frequency, therefore, can be assessed only by taking the highest of these figures as a minimum. Such a rectification of the French rate leads to the conclusion that there are at least 60,000 deaths every year from cancer, instead of the 35,000 suggested by the official statistics.

This is fully confirmed by the most recent records from the United States, where, over and above the government figures, there are valuable statistics available from the large insurance companies. According to Dublin, some 168,000 persons died here of cancer in 1942, and when the various errors just discussed are taken into account he estimates that the number would fall not far short of 175,000.

The latest returns from various countries indicate that cancer is slowly but surely assuming second place on the list of fatal diseases, being preceded now only by disorders of the heart. In civilized lands at least 11 out of every 100 persons living are destined to die of cancer. These are disquieting figures and there can be no doubt that this malady, by reason of its high frequency, represents a menace of the utmost gravity.

Furthermore, an impression is abroad that this frequency, high as it may be, is still increasing and it is clear that a disease already common would become a source of even deeper concern were its death rate to keep on rising. But in a question of such weight impressions are an unsafe guide; we require established facts, based on statistics.

Here again records from different countries lead to different conclusions. Certain among them, like Switzerland and the Austria of bygone days, report a relatively small increment in cancer mortality over the past 40 or 50 years, whereas the figures for others, England, for example, or the United States, indicate a definite rise. According to Schereschewsky the rate for the latter country went from 63 per 100,000 in 1900, to 83.4 per 100,000 in 1920, and Duffield and di Mario found a steady augmentation for New York City from 68.2 per 100,000 in 1901, to 148.8 per 100,000 in 1938.

On the whole, all the figures just cited point to a constant increase in cancer mortality, leaving in doubt only its extent. Yet no problem in statistics is simple, and if any reliable conclusion is to be reached two facts must be kept in mind.

First there must be taken into account the *apparent augmentation*, which comes in part from an improvement of general medical conditions, in part from a wider knowledge of the malady and especially from new achievements in the field of diagnosis. The first factor certainly accounts for the differences existing between the various countries so far as an increase of cancer is concerned. It has already been explained that the frequency with which the disease is recorded depends upon the number of physicians in any given community and the equipment available for diagnosis and registration. So it need cause no surprise that in countries where considerable progress has been made in such matters the frequency curve should rise more than in others that have remained more or less unchanged in these respects. The remaining factor is the increased accuracy with which modern technics, and especially X rays, reveal cancer of internal organs like the lung, digestive tract, and brain. The importance of this influence is reflected in all recent statistics. Thus if with Duffield and di Mario we divide cancers into two groups, those accessible to direct examination like cancer of the skin, mouth, breast, and genital organs, and those that are inaccessible like cancer of the stomach, liver, digestive tract, lung, and kidney, it will be seen that the increase in the mortality for New York is confined to the latter class. Obviously the rise is brought about largely by more frequent discovery, and this explains also why in all statistics the increment bears more heavily on males. It is because cancer in women almost always affects accessible sites, whereas in men it is most often the internal organs that are attacked.

Secondly, we have to consider the *absolute increase* of cancer mortality in relation to the increasing average age of a given population. It must not be forgotten that cancer strikes by preference those who are more or less advanced in years, and that as the number of elderly persons in a community increases the mortality from the disease will necessarily rise. So it was in Vienna, for instance, where between 1923 and 1933 the number of inhabitants over 60 years of age was augmented by 40 per cent, and the cancer death rate by 33 per cent. But there was an increment in diseases of the heart and kidney as well for these, too, generally appear after 45, in the "critical age," when a whole series of fatal diseases begin to assert themselves. The fact that an aging population must suffer a rising mortality from cancer, elementary though it be, has often been overlooked in discussions on the relative frequency of cancer among different peoples. Those who assert, for example, that cancer is rare among Negroes, Egyptian peasants, and certain natives of India, and proceed then to generalize on the cause of the malady, forget entirely that these people die at an early age and so escape the chance of developing it.

Although the aging of populations is now a well-established explanation for the rising cancer death rate, it has been asked nevertheless whether the augmentation may not be in progress because younger and still younger people are being attacked. To understand the discussion on this subject it is necessary to know that certain varieties, such as embryonal tumors, sarcoma, and so on, are more common in early life, but that these are not counted in when a "rejuvenation" of cancer is mentioned. This term refers only to the cancers of adult life, like those of the breast or gastrointestinal tract, which are found occasionally in persons under 30 years of age.

Naturally enough one is always more impressed by exceptional cases than by those that follow the general rule, so when a surgeon or a pathologist has encountered, one after the other, a number of youthful subjects with cancer he is inclined to attribute some significance to his observation, though the succession may have been wholly a matter of chance. In the interest of accuracy, therefore,

Berger and I tabulated the age of every cancer patient at the pathological institute in Strasbourg from 1875 to 1925, but found no change during this fifty-year period.

The rising death rate need cause no apprehension, since it is fully accounted for by the aging of populations and improvements in diagnosis. For the individual, therefore, the danger is no greater than it ever was, since the proportion of cancer patients to the total number of persons in the cancer age has probably not changed to any appreciable degree. But to society the situation presents quite a different face. Preventive medicine has triumphed over infant mortality, the nutritional disorders, diphtheria, and so forth, in brief against those maladies that affect principally the young, and the increased average length of life in civilized countries is due entirely to this success. Adult mortality has remained about the same, and although the infant of today is much more likely to reach adulthood the chances that a person of 45 will live on into old age have improved hardly at all. It is here that cancer exerts all its weight, for, together with disorders of the heart and arteries, it is the chief cause of early death among adults. And it is here that medicine has been brought to a stop. The intensive effort to prolong life has saved people from all sorts of diseases, only to transform them into candidates for cancer.

This would be less cruel to the individual, and better for society, if the cancer age had been raised. As it is, the malady strikes at the very flower of age, at a period of life when, far from having reached the end of his usefulness, the victim is still of inestimable value to his family and to his community. From this point of view the situation is serious, cancer a grave menace. The number of persons afflicted and the amount of suffering caused are a heavy burden for humanity to bear, and the burden will increase as the progress of hygiene continues to lower the general death rate.

What is to be done?

The normal reaction of a man confronted with danger is to fight, and against cancer a fight has been going on now for some years with vigor, and not without success.

One of the main essentials in any effective campaign is knowledge of the enemy. In the case of cancer this is demanded first of all from the family doctor, for he is the advance guard in the battle, yet this wholly reasonable requirement is not being met. All who have taken an active part in the struggle realize that the most pressing need, if real progress is to be made, is education of the general practitioner. He must have constantly in mind the prime necessity of early diagnosis, and realize that his most sacred duty in every doubtful case is to set in motion all diagnostic means at the disposal of modern medicine: biopsy, endoscopic exploration, X-ray examination, and biochemical tests. How much time may be lost by expectant waiting and useless treatment! The golden hour passes, and with it the last chance of the patient.

As for treatment, it cannot be too often reiterated that modern methods are entirely beyond the scope of the general practitioner, and that to employ such outmoded medicaments as arsenic salve, silver nitrate, and other vain measures is no less than criminal.

Against cancer there are only two weapons, surgery and radiotherapy. But these can be applied only in adequately equipped institutions and by experienced specialists, for it is more than a mere matter of cutting or irradiating. Careful choice must first be made of the means to be used, and even with the one finally selected there will constantly arise problems that only the qualified specialist, out of his long experience, will be able to solve. It is for this reason that treatment in suitably equipped centers, such as exist today in many European countries and in the United States, enjoys merited and increasing favor. Certainly it is the method of the future.

Thus first upon the physician is laid the duty of understanding cancer and keeping abreast of all the modern knowledge of the disease. But the general public, too, since it is so deeply concerned, since it fears and censures, should keep itself informed, for a greater familiarity with the disease can have but fortunate effects. On this all cancer campaign committees are agreed, for only so can the general practitioner be helped to discover it in its early stages. To what avail his education, and the building of expensive institutes, if patients do not seek his advice until there is no longer any chance of rescue?

That knowledge of this sort can be disseminated has been proved wherever anticancer campaigns have been organized on the rational basis of education by placards, lectures, and moving pictures. Already there has been tangible success. The proportion of persons seeking help for inoperable cancer has decreased notably, and the American College of Surgeons has records of around 39,000 cancer patients who were living and well more than 5 years after treatment or, in the customary phrase, were clinically cured.

Again, a deeper knowledge of cancer, far from accentuating the fear inspired by this disease, is the best means of allaying it. The fight against cancerophobia is quite as important as the fight against cancer itself, for the constant dread of a disease is not salutary, but accompanied by ill health and perhaps even by heightened susceptibility.

It is always the unknown that is feared, and even the most dangerous enemy loses a part of his advantage when the weapons that he employs are thoroughly understood. Only the medical student, in his immaturity, discovers in himself symptoms of all the maladies he has begun to study. A riper experience with disease restores the poise of the normal man; panic makes way for a reasonable appreciation of danger, dread of the inevitable is transformed into resignation, and there come to memory those physicians who, themselves stricken down by the disease that they knew so well, have proved their indomitable courage up to the very end.

None but the sturdiest of souls can reach these heights, to be sure, yet at least one may hope that fuller knowledge will deliver the public from the unjustifiable fears and false hopes aroused by the charlatan.

Finally, it will be of interest to learn something of what has been done toward unveiling the mystery. Cancer research is one of the most entrancing chapters of contemporary science, one of the most forceful witnesses of the power of invention, of the tenacity and acuity of the human mind. In contemplating the amount of work already accomplished, the patience and self-sacrifice of so many investigators, one will be less inclined to criticize medicine because the last word on cancer still remains to be written.

Then it will be appreciated that the cancer problem is of almost immeasurable extent and concerns every branch of biology. As though it were the head of a hydra, each riddle solved is replaced by ten or a dozen others, always more difficult and always further removed from reach.

In the last analysis cancer seems to be closely associated with the organization of the cell and the fact that, unlike any other disease, it appears under the same form in almost all animal species, and even in plants, suggests the impairment of some mechanism essential to life.

But here we approach a frontier that the mind has tried in vain to cross. The life of the cell remains shrouded in mystery because our poor, weak vision is inadequate to the task, and within cell walls the familiar laws of physics and chemistry are valid no longer. If the secret really lies here it is well guarded, nay there is reason to fear that it may be one of those problems which, in the words of Nicolle, will remain forever insoluble because they transcend the capacity of the human mind.

But although the main road be closed, detours may provide unexpected access. Recent investigations on the viruses and the ferments have made known certain reactions that may be concerned with assimilation, one of the fundamental manifestations of life, and from here may be seen the road that leads to the heart of the mystery. Some day, perhaps, it will turn out to be one of the ironies of nature that cancer, responsible for so many deaths, should be so indissolubly connected with life.

II

THE DEVELOPMENT OF KNOWLEDGE ON THE NATURE OF CANCER

THE first primitive notions on what was later to be named cancer must have come from watching ulcerations of the skin that were refractory to all treatment, for an account of these in an Egyptian papyrus of the fifteenth century B.C. constitutes one of the earliest known references to the disease.

By the fourth century B.C., the era of Hippocrates, considerable progress had been made. Other types were recognized, the physicians of those days having been perfectly familiar with cancer of the stomach and the uterus and able to describe the principal symptoms of the disease in these organs, though their conception was wholly clinical. Of the essential nature of the malady they had only the most confused idea, and all attempts to define it precisely ended with the mention of two characteristics: the presence of a tumor and the absence of any tendency toward healing. This was manifestly inadequate, for there are many conditions that combine both features and yet are not cancer.

To escape from the difficulties of this vague definition Hippocrates distinguished two varieties of process. One was the *carcinos,* a motley group including benign tumors, hemorrhoids, and chronic ulcerations of all sorts; the other, the *carcinoma,* which, by its progressive spread, inevitably brought about the death of the patient.

Galen, A.D. 150, with a still better grasp of the problem, instituted a classification that was truly remarkable. He recognized *tumors according to nature,* such as swelling of the breasts in puberty and enlargement of the uterus during pregnancy; *tumors exceeding nature,* such as the bony callus that unites the fractured ends of a broken bone; and *tumors contrary to nature,* which might be either benign, like the fibroma, or malignant, like cancer.

His classification still holds good, though the phrase "tumors according to nature" has been replaced by *physiological hyperplasia,* which, after all, expresses exactly the same meaning.

Tumors exceeding nature correspond with what today is called *pathological hyperplasia,* an overgrowth of tissue that is always limited, never malignant, and, like polyps, related to inflammation or, like abnormal enlargement of the breasts, to irregularities affecting the glands of internal secretion. Galen's conception retains all its value, for conditions such as these are invariably brought about by exaltation of those factors that normally regulate the growth of tissues. The irritation responsible for the inflammatory overgrowths that Masson calls *hyperplastic tumors* creates no new proliferative influence but merely increases those already present, and the same situation obtains with the internal secretions; the follicular hormone of the ovary, for example, which under normal conditions controls the growth of the mucous membrane lining the uterus, causes hyperplasia of this tissue if present in excess.

"Tumors contrary to nature" is an equally well-chosen term that includes what are now called the true tumors. These are contrary to nature because factors are concerned in their origin that are not normally present in the body, and contrary to nature again because, once started, they defy the laws that ordinarily supervise the metabolism and proliferation of the cells. An example will illustrate this characteristic *autonomy.*

In a well-nourished subject reserve material is laid away in the tissues as fat, and in extreme cases the process ends in obesity. Fat is deposited, too, when the glands that control its utilization, like the ovary or pituitary, no longer continue to exert their proper function. In all these instances the excess adipose tissue can be consumed by the body if for any reason it should be required. But there is a tumor, the *lipoma,* composed of fat that differs neither structurally nor chemically from the normal. Yet its fat is contrary to nature, or autonomous, for a lipoma weighing several kilos will not shrink by so much as a single gram even though its bearer fall prey to some wasting disease; all the rest of his fat may literally melt away, but not the lipoma.

Galen was right once more in his conviction that not all tumors contrary to nature are cancers. They may be either benign or malignant, and the term cancer is reserved exclusively for those of the latter group.

Benign tumors, which are relatively common, vary much in character according to the tissue from which they are derived. Thus there are *fibromas,* developing from connective tissue; *angiomas,* composed of vessels and popularly known as birth marks or port-wine stains; *chondromas,* arising in cartilage; *osteomas,* originating in bone; *lipomas,* already mentioned; and many others. All may grow indefinitely, reach enormous size, and even ulcerate, but they remain entirely localized. They never destroy the surrounding tissues and, once having been removed, they never return.

Galen's principles reigned supreme for two thousand years. The centuries succeeding the decline of ancient medicine added nothing to its classic views, for although the Arabs and the great European schools of the Renaissance contributed not a little to the symptomatology, diagnosis, and treatment of malignant tumors, no fundamental ideas on the nature of cancer were brought forward. Methods for investigating the minute structure of the body were not yet available, and no progress was made in this direction until the nineteenth century.

It was Bichat who initiated the new era. His way of thinking cast a new light on cancer, as on so many of the other problems in medicine. Curiously enough, the founder of general pathology never employed the microscope, depending entirely on the old method of dissection, but while his scalpel busily explored the flesh his mind accomplished an amazing synthesis in perceiving the organic unity of the tissues. Where the ancients had regarded all the various organs as wholly detached and entirely independent, his acute mind was able to see that they are formed by the association and mutual penetration of elementary structural units called tissues that react in the same manner to health and disease even though widely separated from one another. Cancer then appeared to Bichat as an accidental formation built up in the same manner as any other portion of the organism, and thus he arrived at the only logical definition for a neoplasm: "adventitious tissue."

The most astonishing thing of all is that Bichat's work was done without benefit of microscope. *Histology*, or *microscopic anatomy*, the science of the tissues, was founded by a man who, in the words of Dumas, "thought that the microscope could never furnish satisfying results in studies of this kind"!

Nevertheless, technical progress could not be stayed, and fresh ideas began to arise on every hand. Leeuwenhoek had long since discovered microscopic elements in the tissues of plants which he called *membranulae* or *vesiculae*. In 1665 Hooke saw the same structures in cork and gave them the name *cellules*, but many years were to pass before their fundamental significance was appreciated. Only in the nineteenth century were they recognized as the elementary units of all living matter, thanks to the labors of Raspail, Collard, Schwann, and Schleiden.

This conclusion was not accepted without criticism, but in spite of all the objections to "chimerical and unintelligible collections of a sort of monad that is supposed to be the real primordial element in every living organism," the cell theory, thought even by Auguste

Compte to be "little complimentary to our present state of intellectual vigor," triumphed in the end. Today it is a theory no longer but an uncontested and incontestable fact that every organism, be it plant or animal, is made up of cells, embedded in a ground substance of varying composition and amount.

The microscopic examination of cancers by Gluge, and above all by Johannes Müller, showed that these, too, are composed of cells, a discovery that merely confirmed Bichat's view; for if all tissues are made up of cells, then cancer, also a tissue even though an adventitious one, must necessarily be constituted in the same way. It was only their imperfect understanding of the way in which cells originate that for a time continued to prevent adherents of the cell theory from going still further and applying all the implications of this doctrine to the problem of cancer.

While it was known that cells may multiply by division it was not yet realized that this is the only way open to them. It was widely believed that they can arise in the tissue fluids as bubbles, whose walls coagulate to become a cell membrane, and thanks to this erroneous conception the old ideas of Descartes on the origin of cancer from lymph experienced, toward the middle of the nineteenth century, one last resurrection. According to this theory, stoppage of the lymph flow causes the exudation of a fluid that eventually becomes transformed into cancer cells; such was the conception, as pictured in all its details by Lebert.

Yet no reliable investigator had ever witnessed the birth of a cell from formless fluid, and with this failure to prove the occurrence of spontaneous generation the idea gradually began to develop that every cell must be a product of the division of another cell. Finally the doctrine *omnis cellula e cellula,* every cell from a cell, was announced by Leydig and in 1855 adopted by Virchow.

The new belief clarified wonderfully the views on the nature of cancer for it could now be seen that since, like any other tissue, cancer is made up of cells, it can originate only as a result of the abnormal proliferation of cells. But at this point two possibilities offered themselves: 1. Any cell in the body that is capable of multiplying can give rise to a cancer; in other words, normal cells can be transformed into cancer cells. 2. Cells destined to become cancerous are abnormal from the first, carrying over some structural blemish from embryonal life.

Johannes Müller, protagonist of the cellular theory, inclined from the beginning toward the second hypothesis and taught that the disease develops from abnormal cells, veritable "morbid seeds," distributed throughout the tissues. But the first hypothesis was not long in finding its advocates too, and the battle between the schools has caused much ink to flow.

The question is important, for according to his point of view one will entertain radically different ideas on the nature, origin, and cause of cancer. Those who accept the transformation of normal into malignant cells regard the disease as acquired and seek outside the cell for the cause of its profound change. Supporters of the second hypothesis, on the other hand, adopt a more fatalistic point of view in their belief that a person may carry within himself from birth the seeds of cancer, which they trace to hereditary factors or developmental errors imposed during the obscurity of embryonal life.

Neither school is entirely wrong and neither entirely right.

The cell theory, though it greatly clarified ideas on the nature of cancer, was beset by many difficulties in its attempts to explain the variable structure of tumors. Laënnec, already aware of their diversity, distinguished two great classes: *analogous* and *nonanalogous*. Today we speak of *typical* and *atypical* neoplasms. Developing his conception he wrote: "The first type includes tumors that resemble the normal tissues of the body, and there are as many varieties of these as there are kinds of normal tissue. Tumors of the second group bear no direct resemblance to any normal tissue found in the organism."

His opinion was confirmed word for word fifty years later, for it was discovered that the two chief tissues, epithelium and connective tissue, develop each its own characteristic malignant tumor, the first giving rise to the *epithelioma* or *carcinoma*, the second to the *sarcoma*. But this knowledge was bought at a high price. Virchow's dictum that the irritation preceding cancer transforms the connective tissue into a sort of *blastema*, or bud, susceptible of any sort of subsequent evolution, and that all malignant growths, including the epithelial, thus originate in connective tissue, caused a confusion of ideas that was cleared up only after prolonged and laborious research. Finally it was proved that all cells have a certain stability of character that can vary only within strictly set bounds. This is the doctrine of *cell specificity*, to which Bard gave concrete form by completing Leyden's aphorism, *omnis cellula e cellula*, with the words *ejusdem naturae*. Every cell arises from a cell of the same kind.

There may be room for argument on the precise limits of cell specificity, but one thing is certain: The wide variations imagined by

Virchow are wholly impossible, and in no case does connective tissue in an adult ever produce epithelium. Epithelial cancers can develop only from epithelium, and thus we come back to the view so clearly enunciated by Laënnec: "Any tissue may give rise to a malignant tumor, which will generally bear the imprint of its origin."

For certain of them, indeed, the resemblance is so striking that the microscopist can identify without hesitation its tissue of origin; these are the *typical* cancers. Nor is the likeness structural only. It may be functional too, as when bile is secreted by cancers of the liver, or even by their daughter tumors (*metastases*) that have sprung up in distant parts of the body such as the lungs or the bones. Secretion is a particularly striking feature of cancer involving endocrine glands like the thyroid, the suprarenal, the sex glands, or the pituitary, all of whose tumors not only assume the function of the normal organ that they have permeated and destroyed, but actually produce the whole train of symptoms characterizing excessive supply of the hormone peculiar to the gland involved.

Besides the typical cancers there is another type, which varies in structure from its tissue of origin, and sometimes so widely, indeed, that its source can no longer be identified. This is the *atypical* cancer. Between typical and atypical there is such an infinite series of transitions that even a microscopist who has seen tumors by the thousand may encounter something new every day.

The information that has accrued from the examination of these innumerable variants has affected the evolution of our knowledge in three different directions.

First, in a profounder understanding of all the various types of neoplasm. Comparison with hospital records has disclosed the important fact that the structure of a tumor is closely associated with its activities in the body and its response to therapeutic measures, particularly X rays and radium. So when a pathologist endeavors to classify a new growth he is far from indulging in a kind of game to satisfy an abstract curiosity. As a result of his study he is enabled to offer invaluable advice on the origin of the neoplasm, its probable growth vigor, and the chances of successful treatment.

Since his knowledge of finer structural details enables the pathologist to recognize cancer in its incipient stages, long before the practitioner can find it, in fact, microscopic diagnosis holds forth at present the best chance of early discovery. The conscientious physician, therefore, will always employ it whenever there is any possibility of removing part of a suspicious lesion to be examined in this way. *Biopsy*, as the procedure is called, has become one of the most efficacious weapons in the fight against cancer and saves thousands of lives every year.

The accuracy that the histologic method provides for the diagnosis of cancer in man is of course available for cancer in animals, and it is for this reason that the microscope has become an invaluable ally in research. It alone is capable of showing the true character of the lesions induced, and for lack of that proof all the experimental work of premicroscopic days is wholly without value.

In the second place, the microscopic examination of cancer has furnished a fund of precise information on the general nature of the disease and its various evolutionary stages. Its local development, the progressive invasion of surrounding tissues during its anarchistic course, the penetration of lymph and blood vessels and consequent transportation of cancer cells to distant sites, the subsequent growth of these cell colonies in the organs where they come to rest, all have been studied in the greatest detail. Indeed, our entire fund of exact knowledge rests upon foundations laid by the microscope.

Finally, the microscope has furnished some indication of the cause of cancer. By a study of its earliest phases the pathologist has gradually learned to recognize changes in the tissues that often precede it, and naturally has been led to inquire whether these may not play a determining role in the inception of cancer. On the other hand, the structure of certain neoplasms closely resembles that of embryonal tissue, an observation naturally suggesting more or less justifiable assumptions respecting their nature.

Thus by way of reward for his patient labor the pathologist is allowed to pass beyond the realm of concrete and demonstrable fact. Ideas have arisen, tenuous at first, later taking form, to crystallize at last in a number of definite conceptions. Not yet having been consecrated by experiment, these remain only working hypotheses, but even so they have been immensely valuable. If some inaccuracies, and even errors, must be admitted, all hold a germ of truth nevertheless, but their highest merit is that they stimulate research and bring about the clash of ideas that underlies all progress.

For this reason we must examine them a little more closely before embarking on our discussion of experimental cancer research.

III

THREE HYPOTHESES

SINCE the days of Galen, who attributed cancer to an accumulation of "black bile" in the tissues, one hypothesis after another has been formulated, as might well be expected in the case of a malady so baffling. The great majority of them have been mere products of the imagination that hardly merit the name hypothesis, and only a few able to boast a rational scientific foundation.

Yet some members of the first group enjoyed an extraordinary vogue. Thus the lymphatic hypothesis of Descartes, for example, entirely supplanted Galen's doctrine, which, after all, was not so wholly fantastic as some of the conjectures that appeared hundreds of years later. For when it is remembered that methylcholanthrene, one of the most powerful among all the many agents employed to produce experimental malignant tumors, is a derivative of bile acids, one can only marvel that a relationship between bile and cancer should have been suggested more than two thousand years ago.

Following the lymphatic hypothesis came a multitude of other guesses aimed at the body fluids, the great group of *humoral* hypotheses, and when pathology at last turned its attention away from the body fluids and toward the cells the explanations for cancer naturally enough shifted in the same direction. Now was fancy given even freer rein, and there appeared a whole series of gratuitous assumptions whose only basis was speculation pure and simple.

A good example of these is the whimsy of cell fertilization, according to which cancer arises in consequence of sexual congress between a cell of the fixed tissues and a leucocyte or a microbe. "By this anarchistic act," wrote Hallion, "the cell is freed of all control over its further development. The harmonious plan followed until then could not be more expressly violated than by an inopportune and unanticipated fertilization that substitutes for the normal growth impulse inherited from the ovum a generative impetus entirely new. The pact to which all the elements of the body had faithfully subscribed is now broken, and the guilty cell gives rise to a free race that recalls in both habit and origin those species in which the cells pursue an independent existence."

Such a supposition, which no investigator of today could by any stretch of the imagination entertain, may be of interest from a moral and speculative point of view but it contains not a shred of truth, for never has there been observed the slightest indication of union by any of the body cells, apart from those of the sex glands. As for leucocytes or microbes that succeed in penetrating cells, they are there as enemies and not in the role of Cupid. Furthermore, the conjecture loses all sight of the fact that the body cell is not an ovum, and that even if some fortuitous occurrence were able to imitate fertilization growth could never follow, for all the immense potentiality of the ovum is missing.

The supposition has been cited only because there was a time when it was widely discussed and seriously considered, even by investigators of renown. There have been many, many others, less picturesque, no doubt, but resting on such equally flimsy foundations that even their simple enumeration is unnecessary.

Accordingly we shall be concerned only with the second and more meritorious group, already briefly mentioned in the preceding chapter. Of these, the most important are the irritation, the embryonal, and the parasitic, or microbic, hypotheses.

THE IRRITATION HYPOTHESIS

In watching the development of cancers that were easily accessible to examination, those of the skin for example, physicians of the olden days noticed that they rarely appeared in healthy areas but were almost always preceded by chronic inflammatory conditions such as scars, ulcerations, or fistulas. This caused the impression that chronic inflammation and cancer are in some manner related, and when post-mortem observation showed that what was true for the skin applied equally to many of the internal organs the suspicion became so strong that by the second half of the nineteenth century clinicians like Broussais and Billroth were denouncing chronic inflammation as the cause of cancer.

Upon what evidence does this opinion rest?

Let cancer of the skin serve as an example. It often arises on chronic inflammatory lesions such as those associated with lupus especially, with old fistulous tracts leading down to diseased bones, or with varicose ulcers of long duration. Furthermore, it is particularly common on the face and forearms among sailors and farmers, where the irritation of continuous sunburn sets up a chronic inflammation that Unna called "sailor's skin."

In other cases it appears in scars, most often in those resulting from burns suffered long years before. A striking example of this type is the cancer of the abdominal skin frequently seen in natives of Kashmir, who for warmth carry a basket of glowing charcoal under their robes. The burns that so often follow are responsible for the development of cancer at a site peculiar to that country, and to Japan, where a somewhat similar practice is in vogue.

But the instances so far cited by no means exhaust the list. Cancer of the lower lip occurs in pipe smokers at the place where the stem habitually rests, cancer of the penis attacks almost exclusively the uncircumcised races, and, finally, there is the great group of industrial cancers such as those of chimney sweeps, cotton spinners, and those who handle tar or paraffin, or are engaged in the manufacture of aniline dyes, or expose themselves constantly to X rays or radium without adequate protection. Here, again, the noxious influence causes slowly progressive changes in the skin that may terminate in cancer.

As for the mouth, there may be mentioned cancer of the mucous membrane lining the cheeks among those who chew betel nut, and cancer of the tongue, that arises so frequently in areas of leukoplakia whether or not these are of syphilitic origin. Cancer of the esophagus is more common among men than among women on account, it is said, of the irritating effects of tobacco and alcohol. This passage suffers, too, because by reason of its small caliber it is continually irritated by hot or imperfectly masticated food, and the widespread occurrence of esophageal cancer among the Chinese is ascribed to the custom of swallowing their rice while it is still almost boiling hot. At any rate there is a popular and perhaps justifiable belief that very hot foods will cause cancer of the esophagus.

Cancer of the stomach is thought by some physicians to develop almost always at the edge of an old ulcer, whereas others believe such an occurrence to be the exception, and there is a similar difference of opinion over the question whether chronic gastritis, accompanied or not by proliferation of the glands, predisposes to cancer of the stomach.

In the intestinal tract it is the large intestine almost alone that bears the brunt of cancer, for which the explanation has been offered that it is the only segment whose contents are solid and whose walls, therefore, are exposed to the chance of damage.

Ninety per cent of hepatic cancers are found in livers that are deranged by the chronic inflammatory changes of cirrhosis, and an almost equally large proportion of cancers of the gall-bladder are associated with gall-stones.

To the foregoing list, already long, there may be added the pulmonary cancer so common among the miners of Schneeberg, who breathe a particularly irritating dust containing cobalt, arsenic, and radioactive material; and a large number of cancers that originate at points subjected to the mechanical irritation of pessaries, poorly fitting dentures or bridgework, or any foreign body of similar nature.

Nor is this association between chronic irritation and cancer limited to man. Far from it. Comparative pathology has contributed its full share of examples among the lower creatures, two of which come immediately to mind: cancer of the skin in draft animals at sites subjected to friction by the harness, and cancer of the mouth in horses where the bit rests.

All these observations together constitute impressive evidence of a close relationship between cancer and chronic inflammations of all sorts and degrees, and it was but natural to inquire whether these lesions, so different in their nature, might not have something in common that is responsible for the malignant change. To this question the microscope seemed for a time to provide an answer.

It revealed the fact that every injury to the tissues is followed by a state of irritation, in which the cells at the site are stimulated to multiply in order that the damage may be repaired. If for one reason or another the noxious influence should persist the irritation persists with it, and the proliferation grows more and more excessive and more and more irregular. So it seemed only reasonable to infer that if such a condition of affairs were to last year in and year out it must almost necessarily end in cancer.

Indeed Virchow, justly called the father of the irritation hypothesis, insisted that this actually is what happens. Whatever the type of inflammation, be it from burns, soot, or sunlight, the result is always the same: chronic inflammation. And chronic inflammation leads to cancer.

Yet this hypothesis, so plausible, not to say so obvious, served after all but the one purpose of uniting the miscellaneous observations of the practitioner. It was an attempt at synthesis, and as such satisfied the human need of coördinating apparently dissimilar findings into one system. The result, it must be confessed, often pleases and satisfies the mind, but does not make for progress, and if it starts research off on a false scent may be in reality prejudicial.

Clinical experience had brought forward a multitude of valuable observations respecting the cause of cancer, but instead of being submitted one by one to minute experimental examination these were thrown together into a hypothesis. Thenceforth this doctrine held sway, and for fifty years irritation was discussed from every standpoint but actual knowledge of the cause of cancer advanced by not one single step. Only when two Japanese investigators conceived the idea of attacking the problem as it should have been attacked from the first, by long and patient experimental verification of a solitary fact, did progress begin.

The irritation hypothesis achieved such great success, especially among the practitioners of medicine, because it squared so remarkably with the observed facts, of which, at the most, it was but a transcription.

In nearly all cases the malignant change begins in a region modified by chronic inflammation, and so gradually, according to the hypothesis, that even under the microscope its earliest stages cannot be recognized. The epithelial cells can be seen multiplying and giving rise to more and more abnormal forms. *Mitoses,* or division figures, are numerous and the excess cells are heaped up in abnormal arrangement, filling the excretory ducts of glands or forming projections on the surface of the body. The connective tissue barrier that should limit the epithelium is often compressed, and sometimes has even permitted downgrowth of the epithelium. But all this is not yet cancer, though one often has the impression that the malignant change, if it is to occur at all, may set in at any moment.

Precancerous condition, say some microscopists, and the vivid phrase enjoys high favor. Nevertheless, it wholly conceals the agonizing doubt suffered by the unfortunate pathologist that is called upon to interpret a lesion whose present nature is plain enough but whose future course he is wholly unable to forecast. In any case the expression should not be taken too literally. Every day the pathologist sees conditions that he is forced to call precancerous though he knows perfectly well that many of them will never undergo malignant change, for as ill luck would have it there is no way of distinguishing with certainty between those that actually are precancerous and those that only appear to be so. Thus the surgeon, anxious to obviate the development of a cancer in the future, is often hurried into performing a radical and perhaps even mutilating operation for a perfectly harmless lesion. Driven into a corner in his attempts at prevention he imitates Herod, as des Ligneris has so wittily remarked, and strikes down all in his path to be sure of not missing what he wants to reach.

It is in such a situation as this that the irritation hypothesis shows one of its weakest sides. If irritation is the only cause of cancer why should two lesions that appear to be identical pursue such different courses?

Furthermore, the doctrine has been justly attacked for failing to take into account those cancers that originate in the absence of any preliminary irritation, for unquestionably there are such. To this objection its defenders have always had a facile reply: It is too late, they say, to prove the absence of all preceding inflammation once a malignant tumor has developed.

But the most serious shortcoming of all is the failure of the hypothesis to explain why all irritations do not end in cancer. So many persons with varicose ulcers of long standing escape, so many with scars of all varieties, so many pipe smokers! Much has been made of cancers that arise from cavities in tuberculous lungs, but for every such case there are hundreds and hundreds of patients with pulmonary tuberculosis who never develop cancer of the lung. And so with most of the examples brought forward in preceding paragraphs; irritation is always the rule, cancer always the exception.

Thus infatuation with the irritation hypothesis comes of the "hypnosis of positive cases," combined with total neglect of the countless negative ones.

But why should one of two apparently identical lesions become cancerous and the other not?

An attempt has been made to answer this question by the assumption that cancer cells constitute a new race, created in accordance with one or the other of two great biological principles: *selection* and *mutation.*

Selection, as everyone knows, consists in the progressive sorting out, as a consequence of adaptation to new conditions, of types better fitted to survive or multiply. Mutation, on the contrary, represents a sudden acquisition of new characters and their transmission to subsequent generations.

Selection was defended above all by Ménétrier, according to whom chronic irritation is accompanied by repeated and prolonged tissue damage that is characterized by alternating destruction and regeneration. Many cells die off, but those able to resist the adverse conditions acquire an exalted growth capacity and aggressiveness, relinquishing at the same time the activities that kept them in harmony with the organism, now become for them a hostile soil. They grow increasingly independent and their progressive loss of differentiation causes the gradual appearance of new properties that lead by continuous stages from the simply irritated cell, through the hyperplastic cell, to the cancer cell.

But the sifting out of such a highly specialized cell race does not always succeed. Like all selection, the operation is prolonged and frequently exposed to critical situations where a sudden destructive impulse may annihilate in a few moments a strain that has been years in developing. The production of cancer cells requires, therefore, an extraordinary concurrence of favorable circumstances, and this is why they appear in but a small proportion of cases, and as a rule only after a long preparatory period.

The sum and substance of mutation has been admirably expressed in a hypothesis formulated by Boveri, who saw the cancer cell as a clock running riot without a pendulum, a cell shorn of the mechanism that governs division.

The seat of this mechanism is probably the nucleus. When this divides normally its contents are equally apportioned between the two resulting daughter cells, each of which receives the amount required for normal existence. In tissues exposed to chronic irritation, however, there are frequently observed abnormal divisions that end by establishing not two, but three, or even four cells. The distribution of nuclear material will then be unequal, and some of the daughter cells may lack just the mechanism that controls mitosis. But as there are innumerable chances that such a cell will suffer still other malformations, which will prevent it from living and continuing its kind, the sole combination among thousands of others that will produce one able to live and proliferate has only an infinitesimal chance of realization. This is the reason why cancer is so rare in comparison with the many occasions upon which it has an opportunity to originate.

These two concepts, selection and mutation, be it understood, are purely speculative. Each satisfies the need for which it was established in explaining why all irritative lesions do not end in malignant growth, but in so doing each has to present cancer as the result of an unusual coincidence of propitious circumstances. Thus it is made to seem a little like the winning number in a lottery with an infinite variety of combinations.

The hypothesis of irritation becomes, in truth, the hypothesis of chance: during his lifetime everyone suffers lesions that might become malignant, and fortune alone determines whether they will or not.

Such a point of view troubles the mind, for it is difficult to reconcile with the fact that the development of cancer, in spite of all its vagaries, does appear to follow certain rules. Chance also has its laws, certainly, and its introduction as a determining factor for the inception of the malignant change might open the way to employment of the mathematics of probability. No such inquiry into the relationship between chronic irritation and cancer, however, seems yet to have been made, and would be extremely difficult in any case because no precise information is available concerning the frequency of irritative lesions in any given organ.

But other objections to the irritation hypothesis still remain. If irritation and chance are the sole determining influences in causation, why are malignant tumors ascribed to the former most often of epithelial origin, despite the fact that the connective tissue participates in irritation at least as fully as the epithelium?

Again, every variety of cancer sets in at a time of life that is characteristic for it, in the body of the uterus, for example, later than in the uterine cervix. Yet irritative lesions at these two sites do not show a corresponding age difference.

Finally, though the same organs are not involved, men and women are attacked by cancer with about equal frequency, the susceptibility of the genital system in women being counterbalanced by a much higher frequency of cancer of the gastrointestinal tract, lung, and kidney in men. It seems hardly probable that irritative lesions of these organs should be so much more common in males as to account for this unequal distribution between the two sexes.

All these objections indicate that the origin of cancer depends upon conditions much more general than irritation, and that this is not the whole explanation.

As irritation, even in combination with chance, does not account satisfactorily for the known facts, other agencies have been added to supplement its deficiencies. It would be wearisome, however, to enumerate all the hypotheses that have issued from this pastime and only one example, therefore, will be given, drawn from Lumière's book, Cancer, Maladie des Cicatrices.

According to his conception, based on a clinical study of scars, four factors are essential for the malignant change:

1. The slow formation of a scar.

2. Aging of the scar, its cells meanwhile acquiring the characteristics of youth. This bizarre notion of rejuvenescence through senility assumes a series of colloidal changes analogous to those that take place during the incubation of an egg. By them the cells are rendered potentially cancerous, but if they are to become actually so there is required

3. Renewed injury, and

4. Appropriate changes in the body fluids of a nature still in dispute.

The supposition marks considerable progress and, as will be seen on a subsequent page, coincides remarkably well with certain conditions established experimentally by Rous and his associates for the development of tar cancer in the rabbit.

By this conception irritation is deposed from its proud state as the sole cause of cancer, to become only one link in an almost endless chain of happenings, and we return again to the same inevitable conclusion: in order that the irritation hypothesis may be acceptable it must be bolstered up with subsidiary hypotheses, whose number grows larger and larger as we analyze more and more closely all the factors contributing to the malignant change. Finally a point is reached where no hypothesis can explain anything, for each one is at the mercy of facts to which it tries to adapt itself as best it may.

If in spite of all this the irritation hypothesis has reached a venerable old age it is only because the idea was not in crass opposition to the known facts, and above all because no better one has been found to replace it. It ceased to be defensible, however, when experimental research proved that one of its main tenets, the nonspecific causation of cancer, could no longer be vindicated.

It has been explained in the opening paragraphs of this chapter that many varieties of chronic irritative lesions may terminate in cancer. Hence came the idea that it is not an independent, specific disease, but the secondary outcome of a whole series of conditions, differing from one another as widely as possible and possessing no feature in common save long-continued irritation.

Yet when attempts were made to verify this supposition by experiment it invariably turned out that cancer does not depend upon the *duration* of irritation but upon its *nature* and the susceptibility of the tissues to it. By a great variety of methods there were produced in animals chronic inflammatory lesions associated with hyperplasia that was entirely analogous to this condition in man, but none of these ever went on to cancer, no matter how long the process was continued.

On the other hand, the injection of an oily solution of benzpyrene into a susceptible animal is invariably followed by malignant growth, and a similar result can be achieved with a whole series of other chemical compounds, with carcinogenic viruses, and with X rays and radioactive substances, though in most of these instances irritation is negligible in amount, if not entirely absent. Such experiments as these administered the death blow to a hypothesis that had occupied the minds of pathologists for half a century, and there happened in science precisely what happens elsewhere; the pendulum swung too far in the other direction, and chronic irritation, once held in such profound respect, was cast aside without further ceremony.

Wholesale condemnation such as this is ill advised. What the experiments refuted was merely the notion that irritation is the sole cause of cancer, but this by no means implies that it is wholly without influence. On the contrary, there can be no doubt that it does play a part in some instances, and we shall return to the subject again. Furthermore, the observations upon which the hypothesis was based have lost none of their value. The facts remain; only their interpretation has changed.

THE EMBRYONAL HYPOTHESIS

EVERYONE is familiar with the little brown blemishes in the skin called "beauty spots." These moles, extremely common and always congenital, belong among the *nevi,* or "mother's marks," and represent minor local malformations affecting the pigment system. No one worries about them, and if there are any lesions that seem to be entirely harmless it is they. Yet in exceptional cases a nevus may suddenly change its character, begin to enlarge, develop a pigmented areola, ulcerate, spread throughout the body, and, in short, behave like the most malignant of tumors. This striking demonstration of the origin of cancer from a congenital defect has attracted attention for many, many years. There never was any thought of referring the tragedy to coincidence, and physicians, always on watch for a clue, regarded it as an indication of some connection between the neoplasms and certain tissue defects that are the relics of developmental errors occurring in embryonal life.

As early as 1829 two French investigators, Lobstein and Récamier, attributed the origin of tumors to the proliferation of embryonal cells that had persisted into adulthood. Their suggestion, actually the first rational hypothesis on the origin of cancer, attracted enthusiastic support all through the nineteenth century. Johannes Müller, Paget, Remak, Durante, Cohnheim, and many others took it up and contributed original views and a formidable body of evidence that have done much to increase our knowledge of neoplasia. The idea of embryonal origin, though born of clinical observation, received from the very first the substantial support of pathologists. The microscopic appearance of cancer, with its multitude of cells and swarms of mitotic figures, is not without resemblance to that of embryonal tissue, and the likeness must have been particularly impressive in those early years when the technic of the microscope was so rudimentary as hardly to permit the recognition of minute structural details. Furthermore, the enormous proliferative capacity of the cancer cell seemed comparable only to the vigorous growth of the embryonal cell, and so the adherents of this school were led to identify the two, referring the inception of malignant growth to the persistence of embryonal remnants into adult life.

Their source was thought to lie in those minor errors that so frequently occur during the development of the various tissues and organs. In the folding and invagination to which the embryonal layers are subjected, a group of cells was imagined to separate from their fellows and participate no longer in the common aim. But the "excluded remnants" remained indefinitely as such, and if at some later time, and as the result of one influence or another, they resumed activity, this would take an abnormal direction. For in the normal embryo the cells are under constant supervision and their proliferative capacities are spent in building the diverse organs. In the adult body, on the other hand, all restraint and organizing influence are missing, the emancipated cells being free to follow their own bent.

In order to prove this hypothesis it was necessary to demonstrate the existence of these embryonal remnants in whatever situation cancer is apt to develop, that is to say, in all the organs and tissues of the body.

The program was religiously carried out. Many of the findings, it is true, have not been confirmed by a more perfect microscopic technic, but on the whole the yield has been enormous and it is admitted today that there is not an organ but what may conceal embryonal rests. Their enumeration and description would fill a volume, but a few examples may be cited.

The pituitary gland, which develops as an offshoot of the pharynx, sometimes contains inclusions of pharyngeal mucous membrane, and as this membrane gives rise to salivary glands it need cause no astonishment if traces of these are found occasionally in the very middle of the pituitary.

Branchial arches, most fully developed in fishes, appear in mammalian embryos as transitory structures. Nature has arranged to profit from their temporary presence, however, by using what remains of them for the construction of certain glands in the neighborhood, the thyroid, the parathyroids, and the thymus. Remnants of these arches may persist anywhere in the region extending from the floor of the mouth down into the chest and throughout this whole area, too, there may be found vestiges of thyroid, parathyroid, or thymus.

The mucous membrane lining the upper third of the esophagus frequently contains inclusions of gastric mucosa.

Between the vertebrae, or at the base of the skull, remnants may persist of the embryonic notochord, a forerunner of the vertebral column that appears for a time in mammalian embryos as souvenir of a remote ancestor.

Finally, inclusions of suprarenal tissue may be found in the kidney, along the posterior wall of the abdominal cavity, and even in the ovary.

Any of these malformations may be the starting point for either a benign or a malignant growth. Pituitary remnants in the pharynx may give rise to the familiar *craniopharyngeoma;* branchial rests are the source of a variety of cysts and of *branchiogenic* carcinoma; an island of gastric epithelium in the esophagus may develop into a carcinoma exactly resembling cancer of the stomach; and vestiges of the notochord into a *chordoma,* a malignant growth that usually appears at the base of the skull or toward the lower end of the spine.

All these *dysembryoplastic* tumors must arise from embryonal rests, for no other explanation can account for their structure, and a similar origin can hardly be denied for congenital benign growths like the mole, the port-wine stain, and certain fibromas and lipomas of the subcutaneous tissues and internal organs.

A like source is equally certain for a group of malignant neoplasms that develop in young subjects and that reproduce, down to the very last detail, the structure of their corresponding embryonal tissues. Among these are such tumors of the cerebrospinal and sympathetic nervous systems as the *neuroepithelioma* and the *sympathoma,* some growths of the retina, the embryonal *adenosarcoma* of the kidney, and certain tumors of the ovary and the testis.

No less evidently of congenital origin is a group of neoplasms that are often combined with embryonal malformations of various organs. This applies to *rhabdomyomas* of the heart, composed of striped muscle, which accompany malformations of the brain and kidney, as well as to angiomas of the cerebellum, which are often associated with cysts of the pancreas and kidneys.

In the same category, too, are those conditions in which neoplasms are multiple from the first, such as *chondromatosis,* and *neurofibromatosis,* or *Recklinghausen's disease.*

Chondromatosis means the presence of many chondromas, which

in this case develop from congenitally misplaced islands of cartilage. These growths show a preference for the fingers and toes and the long bones, and sometimes become malignant.

Recklinghausen's disease, unquestionably congenital and hereditary, is characterized by tumors involving the entire nervous system, but particularly the nerves of the skin. In a typical example nodules by the hundred are scattered over the surface of the body, causing deformities that in extreme cases are truly hideous. Like the chondroma, these growths sometimes undergo malignant change.

Finally, the embryonal hypothesis reaches out to include a group of neoplasms that lead us still further into the domain of the malformations, indeed to the very frontiers of *teratology*, the science of monsters. These are the *teratomas*, or *complex embryomas*. They appear most commonly in the ovary, less often in the testis, toward the end of the spinal column, or in the chest, as masses of variable size, sometimes enormous, containing cystic cavities in which may be found tufts of hair, occasionally teeth, and a putty-like material resulting from maceration of the skin with which they are lined. The microscope reveals a great diversity of tissues—skin, cartilage, bone, brain, muscle, thyroid gland, intestine, and lung. All are well formed, but arranged in a perfect hodgepodge, as though in a chicken hatched from an egg that had been violently shaken.

Growths like this, which certainly do not resemble anything human, are connected by intermediate stages with a group of monstrosities that show undeniable resemblance to a torso or a limb. These excrescences, hanging from the bodies of their bearers, must have impressed the early investigators as parasitic beings. Indeed they do represent malformed twins, and years of investigation have gradually disclosed a whole scale, progressing step by step from the simplest congenital malformation at one end through teratomas, parasitic monsters, double monsters, and Siamese twins, all the way up to monochorial, or identical, twins at the other. All that distinguishes the various abnormalities from one another is the stage at which the developmental mishap takes place.

The two daughter cells produced by the first division of the fertilized ovum can each give rise to a complete embryo, and when their accidental severance is complete the outcome is a pair of normal, monochorial twins. If the two cells are but partially separated the outcome depends upon the degree of attachment, and especially upon the degree of development that each individual undergoes; Siamese twins, double monsters, or one normal individual with an attached parasitic monster may be the issue. In the immense majority of cases, however, the cells remain united and give rise to but one embryo. The descendants issuing from the few divisions after the first are still able to form almost any of the body tissues but no longer have the power to generate a complete embryo, and if one of these cells should now become side-tracked it will give rise to a teratoma.

As the growth of the embryo continues the cells differentiate little by little, becoming as they do so more and more restricted to the production of one certain tissue. Any tumors arising from them, therefore, will bear the imprint of that tissue, though they often reproduce an earlier embryonal stage with all its inherent possibilities of further development. Such is the case with embryonal neoplasms of the nervous system, the kidney, and the sex organs.

When their differentiation has been completed at last the cells of the embryo have become so highly specialized that tumors formed from them consist of but one single cell type. This is true of most benign and malignant new growths.

The various developmental mishaps and the tumors that may develop from them thus form an unbroken series, at the opposite extremes of which stand the twin and the cancer, the latter being in a sense a distant, simplified, and somewhat degenerated relative of the former.

An extraordinarily vivid conception, this embryonic hypothesis, to which one would willingly deny neither audacity nor amplitude! Yet its imposing façade has always concealed a weakness that has been made more and more evident by the very investigations designed to support it.

The hypothesis demands the existence of embryonal inclusions or tissue malformations, and these have been found, but in such abundance that they actually outnumber the tumors; it must be that the great majority of them never undergo malignant change. Furthermore, moles bear witness before all the world that the hypothesis is untrustworthy, for there is hardly a person without one; yet for every mole that ends in cancer there are tens of thousands that do not.

Hence the embryonal hypothesis encountered exactly the difficulties that harassed the irritation hypothesis. Each incriminated one single factor, which critical examination showed to be operative in but a small proportion of cases. Each, too, employed the same subterfuge; when one cause alone turned out to be inadequate a second was added, or even a third.

To support the embryonal hypothesis Cohnheim resorted to irritation, and his logic seemed reasonable and convincing. Of itself, neither an embryonal rest nor an irritative lesion will undergo malignant change, but when chronic inflammation acts on such a remnant it arouses all the forces latent there and drives the cells to unrestricted proliferation. Thus was it hoped, by combining these two hypotheses, to reconcile the apparently discordant facts upon which they had been founded.

Merely to spin hypotheses, however, is not enough. Nothing is easier than to conjure up all sorts of intricate combinations, but they must then be verified by clinical observation and experiment and it was here that the embryonal hypothesis, even as modified by Cohnheim, came to grief. Nor is it a cause for surprise that the substitution of theory for facts should have led to a deplorable confusion of ideas.

It is true that embryonal cells do somewhat resemble cancer cells in appearance, but the two are entirely different in nature. For whereas the proliferative vigor of the former gradually flags as they differentiate to form normal tissues, their malignant prototypes continue to multiply indefinitely and end at last in anarchy and ruin.

But, it may be said, in the embryo growth is restrained by controlling and directing influences; in the body of the adult, where these are missing, the embryonal cell might behave quite differently. Experiment does not confirm the objection. Embryonal tissues in all stages of development have been inoculated into countless adult animals, and always with the same outcome; they never changed their character, but continued to act as they do in the embryo, growing for a time but ending as mature tissues. Sometimes cysts were obtained, sometimes tumors comparable to teratomas, cancer only in highly exceptional cases.

Again, it must not be thought that the cells of embryonal rests preserve their undeveloped character indefinitely, for they do not. On the contrary, they generally differentiate and assume the features of adult cells. Salivary gland cells in the pituitary, for example, or suprarenal cells included within the kidney, are no more immature than their fellows in a normal salivary or suprarenal gland. The only abnormal thing about them is their location; they are not where they belong, and that is all.

Finally, the belief that cancer requires for its inception a combination of chronic irritation and an embryonal rest was proved to be wholly unwarranted by the discovery that cancer of the skin in the mouse can be produced at any site whatsoever by painting with tar. Now as no one would have the hardihood to maintain that embryonal remnants are as widely distributed as all that, cancer unquestionably can arise in their absence.

One last effort to save the embryonal hypothesis was made by Ribbert. He insisted that abnormally situated cells are not under the same circulatory and nervous influences as their normal prototypes, hence are already more or less independent and descending constantly further and further in the direction of complete autonomy, or cancerization. With this conception he sought to harmonize the principles of the irritation hypothesis with those of the embryonal, for according to his notion inflammation causes misplacement and separation such as characterizes the cells of embryonal rests.

But Ribbert's modification met the very obstacles encountered by Cohnheim's original conception. If cell isolation really is the cause of malignant growth, why do only a few of these tissue derangements, either congenital or acquired, become cancerous? Besides, recent experimental research declares the interpretation erroneous. Cells cultivated outside the body are withdrawn from all nervous influence and thus fulfill perfectly all the conditions laid down by Ribbert, yet connective tissue has been grown in this way for more than ten years without its cells becoming malignant; when transplanted back into an animal they act like normal cells.

The embryonal hypothesis, having failed ignominiously to account for all cancer, met the fate of the irritation hypothesis, and for precisely the same reason. Both made the mistake of generalizing too freely and of interpreting as principal causes those that are certainly but second or third in importance.

Nevertheless the facts upon which the embryonal hypothesis was based cannot be gainsaid, and any explanation that is to hold at all must take them into account. All attempts at interpretation aside, they are as follows. There occur:

1. Simple malformations. These include such defects as suprarenal rests in the kidney or vestiges of embryonal organs like the branchial cyst, which resemble normal tissues in appearance and show no inclination toward abnormal growth. In common with any of the body tissues they may give rise to cancer, but they are not predestined to the malignant change.

2. Tumor-like malformations. These have a tendency to abnormal growth, more or less pronounced as the case may be, that results in simple lesions like the mole or in true tumors like chondromas or the neurofibromas of Recklinghausen's disease. In this group there may be seen every possible variety of proliferation. Sometimes it stops short after a certain period, sometimes it continues for years.

Removal of the tumor is often followed by a recurrence with definitely higher growth capacity. Slowly or abruptly some of these lesions undergo malignant change, giving rise to such neoplasms as chondrosarcoma, neurosarcoma, or nevus cancer.

3. Malformations that inevitably terminate in cancer. A typical example of this group is *xeroderma pigmentosum*, a congenital disease that is characterized by a curious sensitivity of the skin to sunlight. The face, neck, forearms, and hands are covered with pigmented spots resembling freckles, which leave behind them areas of scaly and thickened skin that eventually grow out as warty protuberances to end at last in cancer. The most interesting thing about this disease is the impetus given by sunlight, for the malignant change is almost certainly caused by that alone. Another representative of the group is a proliferative lesion of the supporting tissue of the brain, the *neuroglia*, that extends to its covering membranes, the *meninges*. This process, called by Oberling *meningoencephalic gliosis*, affects by preference the region of the cerebellum and the optic nerves, and probably always terminates in the brain tumor known as *glioma*.

4. Malformations that are malignant from the first. Here belong certain neoplasms of the central nervous system (the *neuroepithelioma* and the *neurospongioma*), of the retina, of the sympathetic nervous system, of the kidney (*adenosarcoma*), of striped muscle (*rhabdomyoma*), and of the sex glands. In some of these the malignant transformation has already occurred during fetal life, as in the congenital tumors recently described by H. Gideon Wells.

Such are the facts. We shall see later how far our present knowledge will carry their interpretation.

THE MICROBIC OR PARASITIC HYPOTHESIS

When Pasteur revolutionized medicine toward the end of the nineteenth century in showing that disease can be caused by the infinitely small, his discoveries instituted a swift and momentous advance. One disease after another gave up its secret in the form of a specific microbe, and the problem of cancer seemed on the eve of solution. Vehement hope animated all those laboratories where its microbe, in turn, was being feverishly sought, and for a few years the scientific world held its breath. Success was announced, then denied, and the net result was bitter disappointment.

In 1896 Rappin inaugurated what was to become an endless series of short-lived discoveries, with a diplococcus isolated from cancer. Its inoculation produced results that were variable but all disappointing, for the lesions that it set up in the livers of rabbits were certainly infectious rather than neoplastic, yet with a tenacity that might have been better applied he pursued the study of his microbe for forty years without contributing the slightest proof that it could initiate a malignant new growth.

The bacillus described by Scheurlen in 1887 started a furious battle over priority, but the dispute was for nothing after all since his microbe was soon identified as a harmless inhabitant of the skin.

The *Micrococcus neoformans* of Doyen (1901) enjoyed its moment, thanks to the publicity accompanying its introduction and the renown and guarantees of its sponsor, for Doyen believed it to be the cause not only of cancer but of all benign and malignant tumors. In reality, it was but a common staphylococcus.

And so could be continued a list of investigators by the dozen and an equally long list of microbes, but the same performance invariably took place. Cancers were examined for microorganisms, one was found, and if it were the same microbe several times in succession it was confidently hailed as the cause of cancer. Naturally cultures were not forgotten, nor animal inoculations, which sometimes gave rise to infectious lesions that were interpreted as cancer by investigators who were more content than competent. Then the die was cast! The press, rashly informed of the findings, began its probing, and a veritable bedlam now surrounded the poor inquirer who thought that at long last he had discovered the cause. Serious discussion was no longer possible. Those who denied the malignant nature of the lesions induced by the organism were accused of obduracy, and some investigators, indeed, went so far as to risk their scientific future by defending against all comers what they conceived to be their great discovery.

Such a spectacle was presented hardly eight years ago, when it was announced to an astonished world that tomatoes are the cause of cancer. Not only announced but proved! For the injection of tomato juice into the peritoneal cavities of rats was said to have been promptly followed by sarcomas, and photomicrographs were offered in support of the assertion. Well, it was difficult to incriminate such a common article of diet, so a microorganism was sought, and as though by magic one appeared: an inoffensive bacillus of the subtilis group that everyone carries in his skin. But there, it was said, were the proofs; this microbe, isolated from tomato juice, had been obtained in pure culture, and produced sarcoma when inoculated into rats. No one, of course, was able to confirm these experiments and both tomato and subtilis were thereupon restored to favor, but neither has anyone ever discovered how these "tomato sarcomas" were produced.

Such things have happened periodically, and no doubt will continue to happen, and it is really hard to say whether one should be more surprised at the tenacity with which inquiries of this sort are carried on despite all the evidence, or at the artless credulity of some investigators. Nearly every organism advanced as the cause of cancer has turned out to be a familiar and harmless inhabitant of the skin or mucous membranes, and not a single one, whether isolated from man or from the lower animals, has ever elicited a genuine neoplasm. The only exceptions are certain plant tumors, caused by a microorganism (*Bacillus tumefaciens*) isolated and described by Erwin F. Smith.

How is it, then, that microbes are so often recovered from cancers? Because when these ulcerate they become easily accessible to germs from without, which find in their ragged, necrotic tissue an ideal soil upon which to grow and multiply. Even tumors that have not ulcerated readily become infected by way of the circulation, for at one time or another microorganisms are apt to enter the blood stream, usually from the intestine. Such an occurrence is without consequence in a normal person for these invaders are rapidly destroyed and eliminated, but the fragile vessels of a cancer may allow them to pass through and into a tissue that is especially favorable for their growth. Thus any microbe discovered in a tumor is sure to be the result of secondary infection.

Besides germs, innumerable other microorganisms have been found in malignant neoplasms: yeasts of all sorts, including blastomycetes and saccharomycetes, and even protozoa like the rhizopods and spirochetes. Many investigators, finally, have described cell inclusions, which they interpreted as protozoa and held responsible. Such were the "coccidia" of Darier, the roundish or sickle-shaped bodies of Sawtschenko, the *Histosporidium carcinomatosum* of Feinberg, and others by the dozen. An enormous literature on this subject has accumulated, but none of the alleged organisms has been able to survive criticism, all having been recognized eventually as artefacts due to the degeneration of nucleus or cytoplasm.

When the microbic hypothesis had been proved untenable because no causative organism could be demonstrated, attempts to support it by indirect proof began. But even before the days of bacteriology arguments favoring the contagious nature of cancer had been advanced—its transmission by contact, its frequent occurrence in certain houses or in certain neighborhoods, and so on, and as these have always made a vivid impression on the public it will be worth while to devote a little time to their examination.

If cancer really were contagious it might be expected to attack frequently nurses, surgeons, and pathologists, all of whom come into daily contact with it yet without taking any special precautions. But it is no more common among them than among the members of any other profession, nor does it spread through the patient's family as may tuberculosis and other truly infectious diseases.

Much has been made of *cancer à deux*, that is to say, cancer of the penis and uterine cervix in husband and wife. But the very fact that such cases are published testifies to their rarity, and this in itself is significant when the frequency of cervical cancer is taken into account. One must beware of the hypnosis induced by exceptional cases; and observations supporting the idea that cancer is contagious are always exceptional. Gathered together into an article, often collected without much care in regard to the authenticity of the alleged facts, they may be imposing, but they are mere coincidences with a frequency no greater than can be accounted for easily by chance. This has been fully demonstrated by Lumière and his associates for "cancer houses," a controversial subject for almost a hundred years. Every once in a while terror is aroused by the report of a dwelling with a high cancer mortality, and some authors have broadened their observations to include entire districts, referring cancer houses and cancer streets to the water table, to subterranean streams, or to any other factor possible or imaginable. This is all nonsense, as the following facts will show.

Deaths from cancer are never uniformly distributed and, as is invariably the case when chance intervenes, there will be a series of negative cases on the one hand and an accumulation of positive ones on the other, houses where no cancer deaths have occurred and houses where there have been several. The important thing in trying to assess the significance of such reports is not to be led astray by the positive cases but to remember the negative ones also, taking as a basis for calculation the largest possible number of houses. By so doing Lumière and his group found that the percentage of cancer houses recorded for several communities corresponded precisely with that to be confidently expected as a result of pure chance.

This is true, also, of the "cancer cages" reported from several laboratories, and especially by Borrel. In observing colonies of mice where the same animals were kept always in the same cages, these investigators were impressed by the occurrence of cancer among the denizens of some boxes and not of others. Obviously, however, this is identical with the question of cancer houses. So long as only small numbers are available, 1,000 or even 10,000 mice, chance may result in uneven distribution and highly impressive coincidences, but as the population increases it becomes clearer and clearer that these are referable to chance alone.

Thus there is neither direct nor indirect proof for the microbic origin of cancer. But besides microbes there are other infectious agents, some smaller, like the viruses and some, like the macroparasites, larger. For many years none was considered seriously as a cause, no distinction was drawn between microbic origin and infectious origin in general, and eventually both of these were rejected in disgrace, a serious error, as we shall have occasion to see.

IV

EXPERIMENTAL CANCER

THE first experimental investigation of the cancer problem was described in 1775, when the Académie des Sciences et Belles-Lettres de Lyon offered a prize for the best essay on the causes, nature, and prevention of cancer. Bernard Peyrilhe, who reported the transfer of cancer from the human patient to the dog, was declared the winner; a mistake, certainly, but a mistake committed in good faith.

What had been transferred was not cancer but suppurative microorganisms, and these had elicited inflammatory lesions that were mistaken for malignant tumors. But who could appreciate this in the absence of all knowledge of bacteriology and microscopic technic, which alone could have exposed the true nature of the lesions? The time for experimental cancer research was not yet ripe, and the early investigations led inevitably to erroneous conclusions. Their authors generally forfeited any chance of success by trying to transfer tumors from man to the lower animals, though the attempt in itself was justifiable, for positive results had been achieved with some diseases such as tuberculosis. Cancer, however, remained obdurate.

Others tried to transfer cancer from one human being to another. In 1808 Fayet, Durand, Le Noble, and Biette all inoculated themselves, but to no effect. Still other and less heroic investigators transplanted into incurable patients, but any success that they described is to be accepted with caution. Only the experiments of Hahn and of Cornil, who introduced fragments of mammary cancer each into the patient herself, seem to have been successful. Perhaps they were, for subsequent efforts, the most recent those of de Martel, have shown that autografts in man very often take.

All the early work, however, was futile. Carried out as it was under defective conditions it provided no foothold for advance, and only toward the end of the nineteenth century was a reliable foundation laid, in Germany by Hanau (1889) and almost simultaneously in France by Moreau.

Hanau inoculated metastases from a carcinoma of the skin in a rat into the covering of the testis in two other animals of the same species. Several weeks later he found tumors scattered throughout the peritoneal cavities of both, similar in microscopic appearance to the original growth.

Moreau transplanted a mammary carcinoma of the mouse to other mice, and here again microscopic examination proved the success of his attempt. But he went further than Hanau, carrying his tumors through several generations and even approaching the question of immunity.

The work of these two investigators was so shamefully neglected that in umbrage Hanau destroyed himself, and before it received its meed of recognition a decade or so had passed.

Then Leo Loeb and Jensen confirmed it, and a perfect fury of research set in on all sides. Borrel, Haaland, Ehrlich, Apolant; before long Bashford and Murray with their colleagues, the famous staff of the Imperial Cancer Research Fund; Woglom, in America, and many others undertook a series of systematic inquiries from which much was confidently expected. Enthusiasm ran high, and the hope that animated these investigators has never been more sympathetically described than in the following passage, taken from Borrel:

"In the mouse the evolution of tumors is rapid, and because of its diminutive size every inch of this little animal, including all the organs subject to metastasis, can be minutely explored, tumors recognized in their very earliest stages, and prepared in their entirety for microscopic study. As the mouse lives but three years at the most and produces many generations of descendants, the question of heredity can be submitted to experimental investigation under definite and fixed conditions. One year of observation in the mouse is as good as a hundred years in man. Cheap to buy and easy to maintain, mice can be housed by the thousand in a small space, and hamlets, villages, and cities of them subjected to conditions the most diverse, so that investigation into the cause of cancer has at last become a reality. Thanks to the mouse no limit need now be set to our expectations, and in recognition of its gratitude the International Cancer Committee ought to adopt as its emblem a mouse bearing a tumor."

His prophetic words have been partly realized, but only at the cost of unprecedented effort and by methods that still awaited discovery, for the inoculated tumor was not long in proving itself inadequate to solve the really fundamental problems. In the meantime, however, work went feverishly on until, within a few years, cancer had become one of the diseases most thoroughly subjected to experimental research. Laboratories were organized in almost every country, where rat and mouse tumors, laboriously transplanted generation after generation, soon came to resemble in this respect the strains of microorganisms established and continued by bacteriologists. Some of these, like Jensen's rat sarcoma, the Ehrlich mouse carcinoma, and the Flexner-Jobling carcinoma of the rat, grew famous and were maintained and studied in laboratories throughout the world, for the behavior of the transplanted tumor turned out to be so capricious that all experiments had to be checked by similar tests on several different strains.

Within a few years there had accumulated an enormous number of articles on transplantable tumors, introducing a number of interesting facts but together with them many inaccurate and contradictory notions that fell into oblivion almost before they had seen the light of day. Altogether, this is one of the most confusing chapters of cancer research, yet certain things were brought forward that merit at least brief examination since they survived to be incorporated in the fabric of science.

THE TRANSPLANTABLE TUMOR

Every transplantable tumor represents a spontaneous neoplasm that has been transferred by successive passages to animals of the species in which it originated. As spontaneous new growths occur in many kinds of animals, transplanted tumors have been studied in numerous species, but because of the large colonies required for work of this sort practical considerations restrict the field to animals that are small in size, low in price, and easy to maintain, like the mouse and rat.

Conditions Essential to Success

For the successful transplantation of a spontaneous tumor three conditions must be met: 1. Living cells must be inoculated. 2. These must be introduced into an animal of the species in which the spontaneous tumor arose. 3. The neoplastic cells must be capable of gradual adaptation to successive new hosts.

Let us examine these conditions more closely.

It was very soon found that any condition endangering the vitality of the tumor cell diminished or destroyed the chances of successful transplantation, and a minute analysis of the influence of various chemical and physical factors was thereupon undertaken. In the course of these inquiries it was discovered, for example, that cold would preserve malignant cells for a long time, but that those of different tumors varied considerably in their susceptibility. The net result of all this work was the conclusion that any graft in which the tumor cells are dead is foredoomed to failure. From this it followed that cancer is not transferred by *infection*, as an infectious disease is transmitted through the microbe that causes it, but by *transplantation*, its living cells being engrafted exactly as a gardener grafts one plant upon another. In other words, cancer is not created anew in each successive host as is tuberculosis in animals inoculated with the bacillus of this disease. On the contrary, there is transplanted a fragment of fully developed cancer that can increase in size only by the multiplication of its own cells and that pursues its course in the new host exactly as in the animal from which it was removed; it never incites the tissues about it to take part in the process.

For a long time this conception ruled, a veritable dogma and chief witness against the infectious nature of cancer, for, it was argued, if microbes cause the disease then cells disintegrated by grinding should transmit it, provided the microbes themselves remain uninjured. Today, however, the idea in its original and strict sense is no longer valid, for tumors are known that can be transmitted by extracts from which all cells have been removed. These are the filterable virus tumors, which we shall examine in due course.

Yet on the whole, and particularly in the case of mammalian neoplasms, the success of a graft depends on the presence therein of living tumor cells. Their number is of secondary importance for most of the graft dies off, the only cells that survive being those at its periphery.

Tumors are generally transplanted by removing fragments, about the size of a rice grain, under strict aseptic precautions and inserting them under the skin of the new host with a hollow needle or a forceps. Those few neoplasms that will not grow in the subcutaneous tissues must be inoculated, according to their demands, at special sites such as the brain, the testis, or the anterior chamber of the eye.

For many years all attempts to transplant cancer had miscarried because investigators were obstinately resolved to transfer it from man to a lower animal, and success was achieved only with the realization that it must be inoculated into the species in which the tumor arose. There are a few exceptions to this rule, it is true, yet even there a closely related species has to be chosen; for instance, it may be possible to transplant from hare to rabbit, or from chicken to duck or guinea fowl.

Even in a strange species (*heterologous transplantation*) success may follow the use of certain artifices such as inoculation at a site where protective reactions are less vigorous, the brain, for example, or the anterior chamber of the eye. The latter method has yielded surprising results at the hands of Greene, who has been able in this way to transfer uterine and mammary cancers of the rabbit to guinea pigs, swine, goats, and sheep, and even tumors from human patients have been engrafted with success in rabbits and guinea pigs. Again, Murphy transplanted a rat sarcoma into chick embryos and maintained it on this foreign soil for a number of generations, profiting by the fact that in young animals the biological characteristics of a species are less pronounced than in the adult. Such a situation is much more easily realized, however, by cultivating cells outside the body in media prepared from coagulated blood plasma and the juice of embryos, a technic inaugurated by the work of Harrison and of Carrel and widely employed in cancer research.

Here there is no need for media derived from the same species, and cancer cells from man, for instance, can be grown easily in plasma and embryo juice from the rabbit. The difference between the body and the media used for cultivation in glass vessels (*in vitro*) lies mainly in this, that the former is able to set up protective reactions. No sooner does a foreign protein enter the body tissues than it is set upon and destroyed by various types of white blood cells, the leucocytes and the macrophages, and as reactions of this sort obviously cannot take place in a culture medium the cancer cells are able to adjust themselves comfortably and without opposition. But this adaptation is never actually consummated, for cancer cells from man grown on rabbit media retain all the characteristics of their species. They use the proteins of the rabbit to build up human proteins, and if transplanted into the rabbit are recognized immediately as foreign cells and just as promptly destroyed.

The first investigator to grow tumors in a strange species was Putnoky, who introduced enormous grafts of the Ehrlich mouse carcinoma into rats that had had their resistance weakened by intraperitoneal injections of lactic acid. The tumor was carried along on this foreign soil for generation after generation, though it must be acknowledged that the conditions were wholly artificial; furthermore, in many laboratories where the experiment was repeated it failed utterly. Yet some time later, having lost his rat-grown strain, Putnoky was able to establish a second one, and recently Nagayo has succeeded in transplanting a mouse sarcoma into the rat.

Notwithstanding the almost uniform failure of heterologous

transplantation many investigators continue to attempt it, and every once in a while comes news not only of success but of fresh tumors appearing anywhere at all in the body. Now when a neoplasm is transplanted into the species in which it arose it is usually this tumor, and no other, that appears at the inoculation site, the host serving merely as a sort of culture medium; but occasionally a different one arises, a sarcoma, say, in the area where a carcinoma was implanted. Here we deal no longer with a simple graft but with something of vastly greater importance, namely, the creation of a new tumor that is totally different from the one inoculated. Such an event, noted particularly in attempts at heterologous transplantation, may mean that during their disintegration the cells of the carcinomatous graft set free some substance, or a virus, capable of inaugurating a new tumor; unfortunately the extreme rarity of the phenomenon forbids any interpretation of the sort and banishes it to the realm of pure coincidence.

So, too, with the statement sometimes made that mice inoculated with neoplasms from the human subject have a high incidence of spontaneous tumors, as though the grafts liberated something that increased the predisposition to cancer. The most recent experiments are those of Heidenhain, who reported that 20 per cent of 300 mice inoculated with various tumors from human patients (carcinoma of the breast, melanosarcoma, osteosarcoma, and so on) developed spontaneous cancer, though this arose in but 1.4 per cent of the controls. But in a second series, where the number inoculated was raised to 2,070, the figure dropped to 8.2 per cent, or about the average for mice that are not selectively bred. It is certain, therefore, that if enough animals had been employed the percentage would have been the same in the inoculated mice and the controls.

All such experiments are quite without significance, and Heidenhain's has been singled out for discussion only to show the necessity for large numbers of animals in work of this sort, where otherwise the result may be wholly falsified by chance.

To accustom a spontaneous neoplasm to transplantation is not always an easy task. At its first inoculation only one or two out of a hundred animals may develop tumors, but when these growths of the first generation, or passage, are transplanted in their turn, giving a second generation, the outcome is generally somewhat better, and that of a third transfer better still. As a rule the percentage of success continues to rise as the number of passages increases, until finally the tumor takes in 60 to 100 per cent of the animals inoculated.

In order to understand what passes in the first few generations it must be recalled that animals possess not only a species specificity, due to differences among the various species, but an individual specificity as well, every member of a species differing from every other member, and especially in certain of his proteins. It is these individual variations that, to the intense regret of the surgeon, nullify most endeavors to graft tissues and organs from one person to another. In this respect the cancer cell is more catholic than normal cells, for it has lost some of its biological differences and so can gradually adapt itself to those constant changes of soil that accompany successive transplantations. In earlier passages a graft will take only in animals that happen to furnish peculiarly favorable conditions, but with continued transfer the cells progressively lose individual characteristics and become more and more adaptable. This, however, is not true of all tumors, for there are some that never can be transplanted in series.

The proof that adaptation really is concerned in all this is provided by the behavior of grafts in purebred strains. When a tumor in an animal from such a strain is inoculated into others of the same strain it always succeeds from the first in 100 per cent of those inoculated, because it has been placed amid surroundings to which it is already accustomed. Under these conditions, all tumors without exception are transplantable.

Thus in comparison with normal tissues cancer is less sensitive in respect to individual biological specificity, and it is just this that permits it to be transplanted for generation after generation. But the property is not confined to malignant cells alone, as was long believed, for recent experiments with mammary fibroadenoma of the rat have shown that even benign tumors can be transplanted in series.

The Behavior of Transplanted Cancer

Spontaneous cancer in animals is very similar to that in man. At first the tumor remains localized and grows slowly, but gradually it attains a considerable size, then tends to ulcerate, and eventually gives rise to secondary tumors throughout the body, an event that marks the terminal stages of the malady.

Transplanted cancer behaves differently. It remains localized, but grows so rapidly as to reach an enormous size within a few weeks, becoming as large as, or even larger than, the animal that bears it. At this stage the host dies, generally without metastases having appeared.

Here we come upon one of the great problems of cancer, the dissemination of malignant cells throughout the organism and the relation of this process to the development of metastases.

The fact that malignant tumors do spread in this way, producing secondary deposits in the various tissues and organs, in itself explains the inadequacy of our present therapeutic endeavors. No method, be it surgical removal or radiotherapy, can hope to do more than suppress the primary growth or, at most, reach also those cells that have penetrated to the lymph nodes in the neighborhood; once these barriers have been passed, no known treatment can stay the progress of the disease.

The mere mechanism by which cancer spreads is well understood. From its very inception the disease is characterized by the exaggerated proliferation and anarchy of certain cells, which progressively invade and destroy the surrounding structures. Wandering through the tissue spaces, they break into any blood or lymph vessels in their path and through them are swept away even to the most remote parts of the body. Then, their migration arrested at last in one organ or another, they settle down and develop into secondary colonies, or metastases.

Looked at in this superficial manner, the scattering of cancer cells and the formation of metastases seem to be a relatively simple matter, but more careful examination of the process discloses some perplexing facts that raise a new series of problems.

As the penetration of cancer cells into the vessels and their consequent dissemination are accidents that occur very early in the evolution of a malignant growth, it might be expected that secondary deposits would make their appearance as soon as a cancer is well established, and certain neoplasms do, in fact, behave in this way. They give rise to metastases so promptly that these attract the attention of the patient at a time when the primary growth has not yet revealed itself by a single sign, and when the most searching examination may be required for its discovery.

Fortunately such tumors are rare, most malignant growths metastasizing later than this and some, indeed, not for years. This can be explained only by the assumption that for a time the cells emigrating from these tumors into the surrounding tissues are killed off there, or at least lie dormant, an assumption upheld by a number of observations.

Thus systematic examination of the lungs after death from cancer often reveals clumps of neoplastic cells, *emboli*, as they are called, in the capillaries but no real metastases; and in the spleen, too, where secondary growths are not ordinarily encountered, these emboli are far from uncommon. Many such cells are certainly destroyed in the course of their migration and others survive but lie quiescent until some circumstance favorable to them permits a resumption of growth. Only so is it possible to account for the appearance of metastases several years after a primary tumor has been removed. In such instances, which are far from rare, microscopic examination generally shows that these secondary growths are identical in structure with the primary, from which, therefore, they must have been derived.

This state of suspended animation, *latent carcinosis*, is clearly seen in connection with transplanted tumors. These do not ordinarily produce metastases, as has already been explained, and yet their cells do spread through the body. Two facts prove it. First, the microscope discloses the presence of malignant cells in the capillaries of the lungs or the spleen, and secondly, fragments of these organs transplanted into other animals often give rise to tumors.

One means of provoking the appearance of metastases or, in other words, of converting latent into *active* carcinosis, is extirpation of a transplanted tumor. The method, introduced by Clunet, has its counterpart in man, for every surgeon knows that the removal of a malignant neoplasm may be followed after a brief interval by a sudden and fatal eruption of metastases in the internal organs.

With Roussy and Guérin I repeated and confirmed Clunet's experiment with several transplantable tumors of the mouse and rat, among which the Jensen rat sarcoma gave the most convincing result. Of 258 control animals, upon which no operation had been performed, only 8 per cent had metastases whereas in animals whose tumors had been removed the incidence was 56 per cent. In a second series, where the tumor recurred after operation and was again extirpated, 82.5 per cent of the rats had metastases. Hence there can be no doubt that ablation of a tumor does favor its metastasis, but the explanation of this phenomenon is difficult, and several factors are certainly concerned.

One of these must be the operation itself, with all that this implies in the way of shock, hemorrhage, tissue damage, liberation of growth-stimulating substances (*trephones*), and so forth. Indeed, this was proved to be the case, for operations resembling extirpation in every respect except that the tumor was not touched also increased the number of metastases.

In the second place, removal of a tumor prolongs the life of an animal, often for a considerable period, so that metastases have time to develop.

But these two conditions do not suffice to explain all the facts, and since Clunet's time there has been invoked a state known as *athrepsia.* This term, which means literally a lack of nourishment, was introduced by Ehrlich to interpret the results of his famous *zigzag* transplantations.

When a transplantable mouse sarcoma is inoculated into a rat it develops normally at first, but within a few days growth is arrested, the tumor is resorbed, and soon disappears. If it is removed while all this is still going on and transplanted into another rat it will not recover; in this second host proliferation stops immediately and the tumor cells die without having shown the slightest tendency to multiply. If, however, the tumor is transplanted into a mouse, instead of into another rat, it resumes growth and pursues its usual course, and after having remained for some time in the mouse it can be transferred again to the rat, where it will proliferate for a few days as before. This zigzag transplantation, mouse—rat—mouse—rat, can be continued indefinitely with no harm to the neoplasm.

To explain this phenomenon Ehrlich assumed that cancer cells, like all other cells, require specific nutritive materials found only in animals of their own kind. Thus a cancer of the mouse needs for its existence something that occurs in mice alone, and it can live for a few days in the rat because a small share of this is brought over with it. When their reserve has been exhausted, the cells die. They are not helped by transplantation into another rat, but when reinoculated into a mouse they find again the materials that they need and are able to continue their growth.

According to Ehrlich, this explanation applies also to the absence of metastases in most animals with transplanted tumors. These proliferate with enormous vigor, as we have already learned, and in their overwhelming growth they devour with a thousand mouths, as it were, specific nutrient until the store has been depleted to a point where cancer cells that have emigrated to other parts of the body cannot find enough. The formation of metastases after ablation of a transplanted tumor explains itself on this basis. As soon as the neoplasm has been removed nutritive substances grow more plentiful in the circulating blood, and conditions for the proliferation of migrating cells once more become ideal.

This point of view finds some support in observations on the human subject, where there often exists a sort of balance between the size of a neoplasm and its spread, numerous and large metastases occurring in connection with small tumors and insignificant metastases with large ones. Indeed there is an old adage that runs: Large cancers few metastases, small cancers many metastases. Moreover, Bonne found it possible to reproduce such a condition experimentally. A mouse sarcoma, inoculated into the subcutaneous tissues, grew rapidly and rarely metastasized, but when it was inoculated into the tail, where dense fibrous tissue prevented it from developing into a large tumor, there was a definite increase in the percentage of metastases.

At first sight the athreptic hypothesis seemed a happy solution of the problem of metastasis, but unfortunately this castle in Spain, so ingeniously constructed, so beguiling, was wrecked by experimental research.

The impressive results obtained by Ehrlich with zigzag transplantation turned out to be not so uniformly applicable as he thought, for they could not always be reproduced by others. Frequently when a mouse tumor was inoculated into a rat no appreciable growth followed, and this was invariably true of the converse experiment, transplantation of a rat tumor into a mouse.

When a mouse tumor dies out in a rat, whether immediately or within a few days, is it really because specific nutritive material is lacking, as Ehrlich believed? To answer this question Lumsden incubated the cells of a tumor in serum from a rat in which it had failed to grow. As they proliferated vigorously in this medium, appearing to find all that was necessary for their existence, it cannot be the absence of appropriate nourishment that prevents the cells of a mouse cancer from growing in the rat. The cause of their failure must be sought rather in defensive reactions set up by the tissues of the rat against cells from a foreign species.

But how account, then, for its initial proliferation, and its entirely different behavior, that is to say its immediate death, when a mouse tumor is inoculated into a second rat? It should be explained that this temporary growth is possible only for neoplasms that are highly resistant and endowed with unusual proliferative energy, and that if these conditions are not met a mouse tumor on a foreign soil will perish immediately under the onslaught of leucocytic ferments and other antagonistic agencies. In Ehrlich's experiments the graft was vigorous enough to resist a first assault, and its cells continued to multiply for a time. Nevertheless, it was foreign tissue to the rat, whose organism always triumphed in the end by establishing a barrier that prevented all interchange between its own body fluids and the intruder.

So a mouse tumor actually does succumb in the rat because of inadequate nutrition; not, however, because the rat cannot furnish this, but because it will not. After the lapse of a few days the cancer cells are famished and in no condition to survive a second transfer to a hostile soil. That which did not happen the first time happens now, and they fall victim immediately to the reaction that the new host looses against them.

Finally, the whole idea of nutritive substances peculiar to a species has been exploded by modern research on the cultivation of tissues in vitro. This has shown that pabulum from their own species is in no way essential for their growth; all that is necessary, in general, is mammalian media for the cells of mammals and avian media for those of birds. The specificity is not nearly so narrow as Ehrlich imagined it to be.

But the characteristic behavior of metastases, their relation to the size of the primary tumor, that is, and their sudden appearance after its extirpation, still remain to be explained.

Generalizations are always dangerous, and in attempting to untangle some universal rules from all the recorded observations one should never forget that each of these is subject to exceptions without number. Every new growth, in fact, has its own characteristic behavior, its own inherent growth proclivity that determines whether or not it will metastasize, so that while a certain balance between the primary tumor and its metastases cannot be denied and nutritive conditions, in the widest sense of this term, certainly intervene, there is no need to invoke specific aliments.

Probably the body regards a tumor as just one more organ to be nourished and proceeds to furnish it with proteoses, lipids, hormones, and anything else that it needs. Sudden suppression of the neoplasm leaves all these at a loose end and so provides particularly favorable conditions for cells that have been dispersed throughout the organism, as when extirpation of one member of a paired organ is followed by hypertrophy of the other. It is a possibility. But certainly there are others, and it will be the task of experimental research to discover them.

The stakes are high, for the problem of metastasis is one of the most urgent of all those associated with cancer, from a practical no less than a theoretical point of view. The observations that we have been discussing are defective in many respects, yet not without their ray of hope, for the existence of latent carcinosis without actual metastasis indicates that under certain circumstances the body can prohibit the growth of cancer cells that have invaded its tissues. Realizing this, we may justly hope that once these conditions are thoroughly understood they can be reproduced at will.

Changes in the Structure of Transplanted Tumors and the Appearance of New Tumors

Transplanted tumors preserve in general the structure of the original, and though they may become somewhat more atypical with continued propagation the loss of differentiation hardly exceeds that seen in spontaneous neoplasms. But in 1905 Ehrlich and Apolant described the sudden appearance of areas of sarcoma in a transplantable carcinoma, and their findings were soon confirmed by Leo Loeb, Haaland, Lewin, Russell, Bashford, Contamin, and many others. Today this has become a familiar occurrence, that takes place always in the same way. In examining the sections of a tumor that are prepared by routine for microscopic study at each new transplantation one suddenly encounters an area of spindle cells in the midst of a carcinoma. This may happen in any generation, Ehrlich and Apolant's first case having appeared in the ninth and their other not until the sixty-seventh passage.

At first there was considerable doubt whether these areas actually are sarcoma, and it was suggested that they might represent only an unusual cellularity of the supporting connective tissue framework, or *stroma,* but further observation left no room for uncertainty. All agreed that the spindle cells proliferate more vigorously than those of the carcinoma, predominating more and more with each succeeding generation until finally the carcinoma disappears entirely and the tumor is a pure sarcoma. The possibility, considered for a time, that some of the cells in the carcinoma assume a spindle shape and so come to have an outward resemblance to sarcoma had to be abandoned because it did not fit the facts.

It was found that purification can be hastened by artificial means. Taking advantage of the fact that carcinoma is more easily damaged than sarcoma, Ehrlich exposed fragments of a mixed tumor to heat or cold, either of which destroyed the carcinomatous portion and left the sarcoma in undisputed possession of the field. Haaland employed a more elegant method, grafting the fragments that he wished to purify into mice that had been immunized against carcinoma; after several passages the carcinoma was eliminated and he obtained a pure sarcoma.

Now these sarcomas are actually new tumors, as such the first neoplasms to be experimentally produced, and naturally they aroused the greatest interest. Two possibilities were at once suggested to account for their inception. Either the cells of the carcinoma react on those of the stroma through the intermediation of some substance like a ferment, or a virus; or, which is equally possible, the sarcoma arises quite independently of the carcinoma, perhaps as a result of repeated transplantation of the stroma. It was well known at the time, of course, that the stroma of a transplanted carcinoma begins to degenerate the moment a graft has been inoculated, to be replaced by a new one formed from the connective tissue and blood vessels of the host, but even so it was proposed that a few of the cells might escape disaster and that their repeated transplantation might favor their transformation into sarcoma.

These two possibilities were discussed over and over again. Bashford, Murray, and Cramer had never seen sarcoma arise in transplanted stroma, and the implantation of connective tissue by others never produced such a neoplasm. For this reason most investigators came to prefer the first explanation, the more so because the development of sarcoma in the stroma of a carcinoma is known to occur in man also.

Since those early days the sarcomatous transformation has been encountered in transplantable adenofibromas of the rat, that is, in benign tumors, by Heiman, and by Oberling and M. and P. Guérin as well. Obviously there can be here no question of any influence exerted upon its stroma by a carcinoma, for these tumors are not carcinomas.

The sarcomatous change is actually much more common in transplantable adenofibromas than in transplantable carcinomas themselves, and in our own experience affects the older tumors by preference; thus we found that of those more than 7 months old at least 25 per cent had undergone this alteration.

There must, therefore, be some peculiarly specific condition that encourages it, but in spite of all our efforts we were quite unable to discover what this may be. And so we come back once more to the idea that the repeated transplantation of connective tissue may be one of the influences responsible.

The whole problem is of the greatest interest, and might well repay a careful reëxamination, in which the old experiments are repeated but in a new way. All these were carried out in animals that were not purebred and in which, therefore, grafts of normal tissue had virtually no chance of success. The results might be entirely different if genetically similar animals from pure strains were used.

Influence of Various Factors on the Development of a Graft and the Problem of Immunity

In the endless search for something to influence the course of a malignant neoplasm transplanted tumors have been almost exclusively employed. But though the experiments of the past half century can be counted literally by the thousand the net result of all this industry has been inconclusive, if not actually contradictory, and disappointing in the extreme, for propagable new growths are not suited to investigations of this sort. None of the information thus laboriously acquired could be applied to man, because his spontaneous neoplasms would resist any measure that might be found effective against transplantable tumors. Their use, indeed, has perpetuated error after error and all for lack of the realization that their growth is highly irregular and subject to large and wholly unpredictable variations. Sometimes grafts fail utterly or, having taken, regress after a short period of growth for some reason entirely unknown. In other cases a tumor develops, but after it has reached a certain size proliferation comes to an end, necrosis sets in, and it disappears as if by magic. Or again, a graft may increase in size very slowly, and only after a latent period that is unusually prolonged.

Such incidents as these may affect the tumors in a whole group of animals, and if these happen to have been treated, suggest that the endeavor has been successful though in truth the result is quite independent of it. Naturally the effort is made to guard against erroneous interpretations by employing controls, and mere common sense ought to suggest that there be as many animals in the untreated as in the treated group, but this principle is not always applied. Often, too, the total number of animals is entirely inadequate to the purpose, and many investigators, besides, have the deplorable habit of reckoning percentages on fewer than one hundred animals. If a tumor should regress in 7 out of 10 animals this means 7 out of 10; just that, and not 70 per cent. The outcome might have been entirely different if 100 animals actually had been used.

All this goes to show that the experimental method is laborious and subject to many errors, and that it furnishes results applicable after all only under the precise conditions amid which the investigation was carried out.

Let us examine first the effects of diet on the growth of transplanted tumors. Here, again, mistakes not a few have been made, but it may be said in a general way that overfeeding favors, and underfeeding inhibits, neoplastic proliferation.

To analyze the behavior of the various dietary constituents animals have been kept on regimens containing almost nothing but the substance under investigation. In such conditions the food is often deficient in general, and destitute of vitamins, so that any effect noticed on the growth of a neoplasm has no relation at all to the component in question but is a result of simple malnutrition. Or, again, some elements of the diet, like the lipids, may be actually harmful if fed in large quantities; here any inhibition of the tumor will be an outcome of general poisoning through their thoughtless administration, not of any direct action by the fats.

As for the proteins, no striking consequences have emerged from their investigation. More cannot be said than that a diet rich in proteins, or even confined wholly to meat, causes no appreciable inconvenience to the host, yet has been asserted by several experimentalists to exert a definite inhibition on tumor growth.

A more rational type of inquiry withholds essential compounds, amino acids of the cyclic series like tryptophan, tyrosine, or phenylalanine, without which the vertebrate organism is unable to manufacture proteins. Since the rapid growth of malignant tissue implies active protein synthesis it was entirely reasonable to hope that its proliferation would be impeded in the absence of these indispensable building materials, but the results of experiments by Coste and others were, to say the least, disappointing. In competing for the necessary elements cancer proved more proficient than the body. It swallowed up all the reserves, and when the need became desperate the organism broke down its own proteins to meet the demands of the cancer, and the animal shortly died of malnutrition. A real biological suicide indeed!

Nevertheless, the idea that inspired these experiments has lost none of its value. It comprises, in fact, one of the few possibilities imaginable today for a rational treatment of cancer, and it is encouraging to see that investigators like Voegtlin are not ignoring it. Some day there may be discovered a substance whose lack will prevent the synthesis of proteins, for Carrel is no doubt right in his belief that man does not yet realize the efficacy of dietary influences in molding his body nearer to the heart's desire.

The effect of the lipids is variable. Their complete absence does not hinder appreciably the growth of a tumor, but certain of them, such as olive oil or butter, tend to do so if present in excess. Cholesterol seems to stimulate somewhat, whereas other lipids, like lecithin, may retard, as may some substances derived from the brain if they are administered in large amounts.

The carbohydrates, and especially the sugars, unquestionably accelerate the growth of transplanted tumors, perhaps because of the greedy consumption of sugar by the malignant cell.

Among the remaining components of the diet the vitamins have attracted most attention, but their investigation is attended by the very difficulties that hamper experiments with the amino acids.

When the lack is only relative the cancer monopolizes the last reserves of the body, and its course is modified hardly at all; when the deficiency becomes complete the body suffers as soon as the cancer, if not sooner, and the treated animals die before the controls.

On the whole, cancer cells seem more sensitive to deprivation of the B group than to loss of vitamin A. In excess, vitamin A appears to have no influence one way or the other, though this condition has been said to favor tumor growth if a superabundance of the B complex be administered at the same time. But as similar results have been described with an excess of the latter alone the precise role of vitamin A is still in dispute. Antagonistic action, also, has been reported, and ascribed to a general stimulating effect on the defenses of the body, and in experiments with transplantable tumors this frequently dominates the scene, for inoculation often fails in the presence of hypervitaminosis A.

Our knowledge, only too fragmentary in the case of propagable neoplasms, proves to be still more imperfect when we attempt to apply it to the spontaneous new growth. Vitamin A unquestionably plays an important part in the nutrition of certain types of epithelium, and it may very well be that deficiency or excess can influence the genesis of cancer in them, but the facts so far known are wholly inadequate and a great deal of investigation will be required to solve the problem. No doubt the situation is infinitely more complex than we realize, and it is entirely possible that the influence of vitamin A varies, not only with the tissues involved but also with the nature of the tumors that arise in them.

The component of the B complex that favors neoplastic proliferation seems to be B_6, according to recent works by Bischoff and Long.

As for vitamin C, little is known of its activities. Investigation is difficult because the rodents generally employed in cancer research can synthesize this vitamin for themselves and deficiency, therefore, cannot be achieved. Excess appears to favor rather than retard tumor growth.

Experiments with the remaining vitamins have furnished no results that are worthy of note.

The glands of internal secretion have been industriously examined. Extracts of the pituitary have in general a stimulating effect upon transplanted tumors, whereas those of other glands such as the thyroid, thymus, and spleen inhibit them. For this reason extracts of these organs constitute a large proportion of the remedies offered to the public, but unfortunately their commercial success is far from justified by their efficacy.

Such a multitude of other factors have been tested that their mere enumeration would grow tiresome, so only the heavy metals will be mentioned. Most of these have been shown to exert a definite retarding action, and intense hope was aroused when von Wassermann and his associates reported that the complete cure of transplanted tumors is possible with salts of selenium. Unfortunately none of the metals, not even this one, has any influence on spontaneous neoplasms.

Transplantable tumors are easily affected by procedures that leave the spontaneous neoplasm untouched. Thus Aschoff found that repeated compression will sometimes suffice, though at others it may have an exactly opposite effect, stimulating growth and encouraging the development of metastases. Or partial excision, which always has a disastrous influence upon spontaneous tumors, may sometimes accomplish the cure of a transplanted neoplasm.

All this shows how hesitant one must be about applying to spontaneous new growths any results obtained with transplanted tumors, and caution is nowhere more necessary than in the case of immunity.

In any group of inoculated animals there are almost sure to be some that will be resistant from the first. There exists, therefore, a *natural immunity* to transplantable tumors, but it is inconstant and often transitory, for an animal that has proved refractory to a first graft may very well be susceptible to subsequent implantation. The situation is different where an already established tumor has regressed spontaneously or as a result of X-ray treatment; here a more lasting immunity appears that nullifies all attempts to inoculate again. A certain degree of protection can be conferred also, and more easily, by injecting large quantities of tumor cells that have been killed by heat or some other agent.

Besredka and his associates employed this method to immunize rabbits against the Brown-Pearce tumor, a transplantable carcinoma that originated in the scrotal skin of a syphilitic rabbit. In other experiments he inoculated the growth into the skin, where it grew poorly and finally disappeared, and rabbits thus treated were found resistant to a second inoculation, even into the testis, a site at which this neoplasm is almost certain to take.

Saphir and Appel amplified the experiment by inoculating grafts of the Brown-Pearce carcinoma into the skin of animals with fully developed tumors. The protection conferred by absorption of these grafts was sufficient to cause the disappearance of the carcinomas already present and even of their metastases.

Experiments of this sort have suggested that an *acquired immu-*

nity may be specific and thus analogous to that elicited by certain microbes or toxins, but the idea became untenable as soon as it had been shown that a similar immunity can be aroused by the introduction of normal tissues. It is clear, therefore, that the immunity is not excited specifically by and against the cancer cell but is merely a modification of the way in which an animal reacts, an activation of the connective tissues such as can be obtained also by the injection of various proteins like casein or nucleic acid, or of lipids.

Nor is it by any means universally effective, everything depending upon the tumor employed. Guérin's carcinoma of the rat, for example, which we have used for many years in experiments on immunity, defies all attempts to protect against it.

Ehrlich endeavored to stretch immunity so that it would cover every tumor at his disposal. He wished to develop a sort of *panimmunity*, which would insure against the development of spontaneous neoplasms, but found in the end that mice refractory to all his transplantable tumors might perfectly well die of spontaneous cancer.

This is the reef on which all experiments with transplantable tumors are wrecked; the outcome is never applicable to spontaneous neoplasms, which alone concern us from a practical point of view. Nowhere does this appear more plainly than in de Martel's attempt to apply the results of Besredka to the human subject. In patients with cancer of the breast he removed fragments of the tumor, implanted them into the skin, then brought about their disappearance by radiotherapy; unfortunately the effort failed entirely to produce immunity, as might have been expected.

Naturally enough the serological changes that accompany immunity have been intensively scrutinized.

When an animal is injected with a foreign protein the organism responds with antibodies that precipitate it and so render it harmless. A horse, for example, inoculated with diphtheria toxin or snake venom develops corresponding antibodies (antitoxins or antivenoms) in his blood whereby his serum acquires the power to neutralize the pernicious activities of these poisons. This property, as everyone knows, is of inestimable value in practical medicine.

Imagine, now, a horse prepared by injections of a cancer emulsion from the human subject. Antibodies no doubt will be formed against the proteins of the cancer cell, and his serum will therefore be able to precipitate these proteins. Injected into a patient with cancer, it might react with the proteins of the neoplasm and so, perhaps, lead to destruction of the tumor. Well, the experiment has been made many, many times, of course, but from the very first attempt, in 1895, by Héricourt and Richet down to the present day it has been consistently unsuccessful.

Why?

Because cancer is in actual fact a part of the body that bears it, and its proteins accordingly are like those of the host. So when a horse is injected with cancer from a human being it is not an anticancer but an antiman serum that is produced.

But is it impossible, then, to prepare a more specific serum, one that shall be directed against some particular organ or tissue? Cannot an antikidney or an antiliver serum be made by injecting an animal with renal or hepatic tissue?

This is the great problem of the *cytotoxic sera*, which has been attacked so often in vain that Roessle concluded his review of the subject with the rather cynical remark that specific sera had been sought against all the tissues and organs save only the umbilical cord, with uniform failure as the result. Gradually the impossibility of preparing a specific cytotoxic serum attained the dignity of a general law, and all hope of success vanished. But not permanently, for such is man that he hopes and seeks eternally, against all and despite all.

Actually, an organ-specific effect can be obtained with cytotoxic sera under certain conditions. Many investigators had tried in vain to develop an antikidney serum by injecting animals repeatedly with emulsions of renal tissue, but Masugi asked himself whether the sera thus prepared had only seemed inert because they had been given in amounts that were too small. He thereupon repeated the old experiment once more, treating ducks with an emulsion of rat kidney and injecting their serum into rats in doses that would correspond to about 1 or 2 quarts in man! The pronounced damage to their kidneys that he brought about in this way has been confirmed in several laboratories.

Meanwhile Lumsden had shown that a specific effect of cytotoxic sera, generally not demonstrable in the living organism, is clearly evident when these act on cells growing in vitro. He succeeded in preparing a serum that selectively killed the cancer cells against which it was directed, but sad to relate it was powerless against the same tumor when injected into an animal in which this was growing.

It is only fair to say, however, that current methods of making cytotoxic sera are rudimentary in the extreme. Future research must endeavor to isolate from cancer tissue some proteins, or other substances, that will be more specific in producing antibodies. Maybe the problem will be solved by the injection of something that can combine with certain constituents of the cancer cell, for modern immunology has shown the possibility of creating in this way complexes against which specific antisera can easily be made.

Apparently there are still opportunities in a domain where the results so far achieved are, let it be confessed, more than discouraging, and even though the investigations of the past few years have done no more than show the way they mark great progress nevertheless. For amid the encircling gloom of cancer the smallest ray of hope is to be hailed with thanksgiving.

This section has discussed some of the findings that have emerged from the study of transplantable cancer. Anyone who has read it carefully will be able to understand them and arrive at some estimation of their true value. But can he picture to himself at what pains they have been collected? Will he realize that for every experiment that yields even the most modest result, alas, fifty fruitless ones or more have been made? Or recognize the years of work and the thousands of animals sacrificed? Those who do know will agree that hardly any other branch of science has demanded such infinite patience of its disciples, or subjected them to such a bitter ordeal. The import of investigations that once seemed fraught with boundless possibilities has diminished before their very eyes. By sad experience they have learned that transplantable cancer is not spontaneous cancer; that facts applicable to the one do not touch the other; that, paradoxical as this may be, an animal into which a cancer has been inoculated is not a cancerous animal. The cancerous animal has produced his own tumor, his body has undergone all those changes that led gradually down to its development, and it is his own cells that have suffered the malignant transformation. The animal bearing a transplanted neoplasm, on the other hand, is but a culture medium for cells that are not his own, and toward which he consequently reacts in a totally different way.

As a result, interest in the questions that transplantable tumors were once expected to solve has inevitably fallen off, for more must never be demanded of a method than it can give. Altogether they have turned out to be a grand illusion, for so little do they resemble the spontaneous new growth that they are utterly incapable of furnishing information applicable to man, or of providing the least insight into the cause of the malignant change, since they were already established from the first.

Begun with enthusiasm, the investigation of transplantable tumors ended in woeful disappointment. "You wish to work at experimental cancer?" said Ehrlich one day to a young colleague. "Do not even think of it. I have wasted fifteen years of my life in that way. Until some fundamental discovery has solved the mystery of life itself our knowledge of cancer will not advance a single step."

Fortunately new paths were soon to be opened up that would refute, in part at least, these somber words of a discouraged man.

THE INDUCED TUMOR

THE transplantable neoplasm failed because it could throw no light on the cause of cancer. An entirely new tumor, a sarcoma, did from time to time arise, it is true, but the phenomenon was so infrequent, so far beyond the grasp of the investigator, that instead of providing a solution it merely added one more problem. Thus it became clearer and clearer every day that any advance was contingent on the discovery of some way to start cancer in an animal, at any desired site and by a relatively simple procedure that could be applied on a large scale.

The first fumbling attempts were patterned after the most prominent hypotheses. Whether from mischance or lack of patience, chronic irritation produced nothing, though later it was to succeed; and those who put their trust in the embryonal hypothesis had little more reason to congratulate themselves. In one experiment after another they injected embryonal tissues prepared in every conceivable way, and while now and then they were rewarded with a malignant growth a malicious fate always prevented fulfillment of the one condition necessary to raise this above the level of pure coincidence, that is, the evocation of such a tumor at will.

Of those unfortunates who spent their lives inoculating animals with microbes obtained from malignant neoplasms it is kinder to say nothing.

As so often happens in the biological sciences, the first success was obtained in a wholly unexpected way.

CARCINOGENIC RAYS

DISCOVERY of the X rays, in 1895, brought with it so many implications for diagnosis that their use became general almost overnight. In total ignorance of any danger the early radiologists handled their tubes without concern, and only a year after Roentgen's discovery the first case of burn, or *radiodermatitis,* as the lesion came to be called, was reported. This is the first stage in what was to prove for so many a long and painful calvary. The years following brought descriptions of chronic lesions of the skin accompanied by ulcers that showed no tendency to heal, and in 1902 Frieben published the first instance of roentgen cancer, in a man 33 years old who for 4 years had used his hand as a test object in the manufacture of X-ray tubes. The carcinoma arose on the back of his hand, and necessitated amputation of the arm.

Other reports soon followed. So many doctors and technicians who had employed the rays without adequate protection fell victim to this misfortune, so many patients were treated in ignorance of danger, that by 1914 Feygin was able to collect 104 cases, and the number was considerably augmented later. In France alone there were more than 100, and for the entire world X-ray cancers could certainly be counted by the thousand.

In man roentgen cancer never appears immediately after the exposure but is always preceded by chronic radiodermatitis, which, in turn, may not become manifest for years; thus a latent period, that may vary all the way from 4 to 15 years, is interposed between the application of the noxious agent and the inception of cancer. The dermatitis involves areas that have been subjected to the rays, usually the hands and forearms in radiologists and technicians, any part of the body in patients who have been irradiated for diagnosis or treatment. The skin of the affected region loses its elasticity and after its glands have atrophied becomes dry, its hair disappears, the nails grow brittle, and in the late stages circulatory disturbances show themselves, in the form of persistent redness together with dilatations of the capillaries and small arteries. As it atrophies more and more the skin contracts, embarrassing the motion of the joints, assumes somewhat the look of xeroderma pigmentosum * and undergoes a profound metabolic derangement. The horny layer is not worn away uniformly as it should be and in consequence warty outgrowths occur that sometimes become detached, leaving painful fissures or even ulcers. It is generally in the borders of these chronic ulcers, or in the areas of thickened skin, that the cancer first appears.

The tormenting pain that accompanies the development of all these lesions, the implacable nature of roentgen cancer, refractory to any treatment and even to successive amputations, make it one of the most horrible of all diseases, a prolonged, murderous agony.

In structure it is an epidermoid carcinoma, but sarcomas also have been observed, and more frequently since highly penetrating rays have been employed.

After so many years the experimentalist had at his command, in the X ray, a means of producing cancer, and it remained only to

* See p. 33.

test it on animals. This was first done by Clunet, who irradiated rats until ulcers appeared and kept these from healing by renewed exposures. Two of the animals developed sarcoma, one 9 months, the other 2 years after the beginning of the experiment; the latter growth was transplanted into other rats and maintained for several generations. *This was the first experimental production of malignant tumors in animals.*

But the experiment must have seemed too complicated to be performed on a large scale, for more than a decade elapsed before it was repeated. Then, in 1923, Bloch described the results of systematic endeavors to evoke carcinoma of the skin in rabbits. With his more advanced technic the importance of dosage was clearly apparent, light exposures having been followed by only superficial burns and very large doses by necrosis without subsequent tumors.

Since that time the question has been studied by a number of investigators and carcinomas of the skin and sarcomas of various types have been elicited in several species of animals. Jonkhoff has produced carcinoma of the skin in the mouse, Lüdin chondrosarcoma in the rabbit, and Lacassagne and Vinzent sarcomas in rabbits by irradiating inflammatory lesions, but because of technical difficulties the X ray has never been widely employed in cancer research.

Roentgen's discovery did not long enjoy its unique position. In 1896 Becquerel proved that salts of uranium emit a radiation analogous in some respects with X rays, and two years later Madame Curie extended his observation to salts of thorium, suggesting at the same time the adjective "radioactive" for all materials capable of such emission. In the course of a methodical search for radioactive substances in nature she discovered minerals that are particularly rich in radiations, and in collaboration with Pierre Curie succeeded in extracting a new element, radium, which provokes effects resembling those of X rays. Again this was found out only by accident, but investigators, forewarned by what had happened with roentgen rays, hastened to institute the necessary precautions and so very little damage was done.

Yet there have been cases of radiodermatitis and even cancer caused by radium.

Radium has been introduced experimentally into the bodies of animals either in the form of radium needles, used for treating human patients, or as silk threads impregnated with its salts. Schürch and Uehlinger have elicited osteosarcomas in the rabbit by inserting this element into the femur, and Daels, and later Daels and Biltris, produced a whole series of malignant epithelial or connective tissue tumors at various sites in the guinea pig and the mouse. Hellner, finally, obtained a sarcoma of the knee in a rabbit by the external application of radium.

It might have been expected that thorium, too, would be carcinogenic, because of its radioactivity; at least the question seemed worth investigating, as thorium salts and other derivatives were being more and more widely applied in medicine for both diagnosis and treatment.

In experiments on several species of animals with *thorotrast,* a colloidal preparation of thorium dioxide that is particularly rich in the element, Roussy, M. Guérin, and I obtained entirely conclusive results in the rat. The injection of a suitable dose under the skin or into the peritoneal cavity was regularly followed after 9 to 14 months by the appearance of sarcoma. With smaller amounts the number of tumors decreased and the latent period increased; thus with one-tenth of the usual dose sarcomas arose in only 50 per cent of the animals and not until after 14 to 24 months. Selbie has confirmed these observations by eliciting sarcomas with thorotrast in the rat and the mouse, and Foulds has been equally successful. Thirty-seven months after he had introduced it into the mammary glands of 9 guinea pigs, 4 were found to have either carcinoma or sarcoma; 3 of these growths were transplantable, especially the carcinoma, which was carried through 15 generations. Recently Andervont and Shimkin have reported sarcomas obtained by the subcutaneous injection of thorotrast into mice.

The carcinogenic activity of thorium, thus amply demonstrated, is unusual in several ways. It seems limited to certain species, for we saw no tumors arise in the rabbit and the chicken, though they were kept under observation a long time. Moreover, in susceptible species the effect is limited to certain cells. In the rat only the fibroblasts of the connective tissue are affected; we never produced a tumor of the reticuloendothelial cells in the liver, the spleen, or the bone marrow, though it is these elements almost exclusively that store thorium in the body and they were literally stuffed with it.

These experiments have found sad confirmation among those who make luminous dials for timepieces. The paint, a mixture of zinc sulfate and salts of mesothorium or radium, is applied with fine brushes that the girls used to draw to a point in their mouths. In so doing they absorbed small quantities of radioactive material that were retained in the body, especially by the reticuloendothelial cells of the bone marrow, and Martland has reported the occurrence in these girls of osteosarcomas involving the ribs, the bones of the skull and pelvis, or almost any other part of the skeletal system, after from 6 to 9 years, even in some who had long since abandoned all contact with the radioactive material.

Of late, too, osteosarcomas have been evoked with thorium compounds in the rabbit by Uehlinger and Schürch, Sabin and her associates, and others.

The conclusion to be drawn from these experiments and observations is that all radioactive substances are carcinogenic. They may be more effective or less, their activities may be limited to certain cells, their latent period may be long, but the power is there, and it behooves the physician to remember.

But X rays and those from the various radioactive substances are not unique in their carcinogenicity, as the earlier workers believed. From these radiations there runs an unbroken series through the ultraviolet rays, then the visible spectrum, all the way to the infrared, or heat, rays. All are manifestations of electromagnetic energy, differing only in wave length, and their physical, chemical, and biological properties have many traits in common. It would be curious indeed, therefore, if such a fundamental characteristic as carcinogenic activity were limited to a few only, and fact confirms the suspicion. Every one of them is effective.

In the section on irritation there were mentioned a number of convincing illustrations of the carcinogenic power of sunlight, such as the relative frequency of cancer of the skin among those who pass their lives in the open air, and limitation of the neoplasms to exposed parts of the body. Xeroderma pigmentosum is an almost experimental demonstration, for here is a congenital affection that reveals itself by an abnormal sensitivity of the skin to sunlight, and whose lesions appear only on exposed areas, to terminate inevitably in cancer.

Experimental proof of the carcinogenic activity of ultraviolet rays from a mercury-vapor lamp has been furnished for rats and mice by Findlay; Wahlgren; Huldschinsky; Herlitz, Jundell, and Wahlgren; Putschar and Holtz; Roffo; Grady, Blum, and Kirby-Smith; Rusch and Baumann; and Beard, Boggess, and von Hamm. The tumors, which often arise in considerable number about the eyes and on the ears, snout, and paws are benign, warty outgrowths (papillomas), carcinomas, or sometimes sarcomas.

But it is not necessary to use an artificial source. Sunlight alone will suffice, as Roffo proved a few years ago with an almost disconcertingly simple technic; he merely exposed white rats to the sun for several hours each day. Naturally this had often been tried before, but the white rat, in common with other albinos, bears sunlight badly and all the experiments had been prematurely ended by the death of the few animals employed.

To escape this difficulty Roffo started with 600 rats, which were placed in the sun for 5 hours every day over a period of 7 to 10 months. Among 235 survivors 70 per cent developed carcinoma or sarcoma in hairless areas like the ears, eyelids, snout, and paws. The growths were often multiple, and it was not rare to find both varieties in one animal.

Light rays lead logically to heat rays. Here we are on familiar ground, for preceding pages have acquainted us with the cancer that originates in the scars of burns, only now this fact presents itself in a new light. Immediately it falls into line with a whole series of others and we see clearly why not all scars, but only those from burns, are predisposed to the malignant change. The cell damage produced by heat rays must be of a specific nature, and must resemble that caused by the other radiations. Another fact, too, becomes more intelligible, namely, the long interval separating the formation of the scar and the appearance of the tumor. As wave length increases the biological activity of the various radiations falls gradually from its highest level in the X rays, with their very short waves; carcinogenic activity probably falls with it, and experiments with X rays and with thorotrast show that diminished carcinogenicity entails a smaller number of tumors, together with an augmentation of the latent period.

In the case of visible light this relationship is even more evident. A protracted exposure is required, in man at any rate, for the neoplasms do not appear until toward the end of a long life, and the negative cases are many.

For cancers in the scars of burns the latent period becomes enormously long-drawn-out, and it has been recognized for years that it is not the age of the subject but of the scar that matters. The average time necessary seems to lie between 20 and 30 years, though intervals much longer have often been noted, as, for example, in a case reported by Bang where 65 years elapsed between burn and cancer.

It may be concluded from all this that every form of electromagnetic radiation, from the X ray down to the limits of the infrared, is endowed with carcinogenic powers.

How do they work?

The answer, though fraught with importance for the problem of cancer, has not yet been given, and there is nothing save conjecture to offer. But one fact at least is well established; the development of cancer is a result of some action exerted by the rays on the cell.

The process is complicated, involving particularly the nuclear chromatin, where the effect may be immediately apparent in the form of a degenerative change that is soon followed by cell death. Such an outcome is observed when especially sensitive cells like sex cells or those of the embryo, the lymphoid tissues, or certain malignant tumors are treated with sufficient doses of X rays. With small amounts lesions less severe, less generalized, and not of a nature to threaten the life of the cell are elicited, but again it is the chromosomes that suffer, certain parts of them being so damaged that they can no longer participate in cell division and are finally eliminated, with inimical consequences more often than not. Or less serious modifications may occur, such as displacement, abnormal splitting, or inversion. Finally, Henshaw has described the emergence of supplementary asters at the moment of cell division, with multipolar mitoses and unequal partition of chromatic material as a natural result.

When it is recalled that hereditary characteristics are linked to the genes, the component parts of the chromosomes, there will be no difficulty in imagining how gravely any of these modifications may concern the implicated cells. Very often their descendants perish, the few that do escape disaster showing more or less pronounced abnormalities that, since they are hereditary, are transmitted to following generations. These irregularities are called mutations.

In sex cells the X ray produces mutations with the greatest of ease. The extensive experiments of Muller and others with Drosophila, the vinegar, or fruit, fly, have shown that in irradiated eggs they are 150 times more frequent than in normal ones, that the resulting variations are generally regressive in type, and that many of the larvae are not viable.

On somatic cells, that is, cells other than those of the sex organs, radiation may act in the same way, creating new races, and it is conceivable that one of these might be a race of cancer cells. This supposition is attractive, the more so because it was to multipolar mitoses that Boveri, whose hypothesis has been already discussed, attributed a predominant role in the genesis of cancer. Hence X-ray cancer would be the product of a somatic mutation.

A beguiling conception, certainly, but unproved, and one that has struggled against a number of difficulties. If cancerization is the effect of a simple mutation, brought about by direct action of the rays, it is hard to account for the relationship between the nature and amount of the radiation, on the one hand, and the duration of the latent period and percentage of cancer induced on the other. And how explain the selective action of thorium on the fibroblasts of the rat while other cells, though in much more intimate contact with the carcinogenic agent, escape unharmed? And why has it never been possible to bring about the malignant change by irradiating cells in vitro?

All this seems to indicate that the process of cancerization is in reality much more complex. Furthermore, the rays act not only on the nucleus but affect certain regions in the cytoplasm as well, and increase the permeability of the cell membrane, to say nothing of modifying radically the circulation and with it the whole metabolism of the exposed tissues.

In short, while irradiation is known to evoke a multitude of changes in the cells and tissues, not one of them elucidates the innermost mechanism of the malignant change.

PARASITES AS A CAUSE OF CANCER

In examining the mummies of those who lived 1,250 to 2,000 years before our era, Sir Armand Ruffer was astonished to find repeatedly the eggs of *Schistosomum haematobium*, or *Bilharzia*, as it is more generally called. Thus the disease bilharziasis, widely prevalent in Egypt today, must have been endemic there for some 4,000 years.

Its cause, a small worm, lives in the veins about the bladder and rectum, depositing its eggs there in such abundance as to obstruct the smaller of these blood vessels. The ensuing circulatory difficulties cause some of them to rupture, the eggs find themselves free in the tissues, and before very long reach the bladder or the rectum, whence they are discharged from the body. The passage of successive lots through the mucous membrane lining these cavities sets up a violent and constantly repeated inflammatory reaction that eventually becomes chronic, and that may end in cancer.

Unquestionable cases of the sort were described in 1888 by Virchow, and soon afterward by others, and systematic investigations since then have shown that cancer attacks about 5 per cent of all persons with bilharziasis, a rather large number in view of the frequency of the disease.

To these bilharzial cancers of the bladder or rectum may be added a cancer of the liver, occurring in man as a consequence of infestation with *Opisthorchis felineus* and first described by Askanazy in 1900.

These facts have not received due recognition. The classic infection hypothesis ignored them, imagining as the cause of cancer a microbe or protozoon or, in other words, an organism of very small size in comparison with the cell that it was supposed to infect. The possibility of a larger parasite, belonging to a higher species, was never seriously taken into consideration and it is not surprising, therefore, that Borrel's first communications on a sarcoma in the wall of a parasitic cyst of the rat's liver should have fallen flat. But no neglect could dampen his ardor, and with all his characteristic enthusiasm he threw himself into a search for parasites in tumors. Other rat sarcomas were discovered, identical with the first and all in the walls of cysts enclosing a *Cysticercus fasciolaris*, the larval form of a cat tapeworm, *Taenia crassicollis*. Acarids, or mites, were found in the milk ducts about mammary cancers in mice and another, *Demodex folliculorum*, a common inhabitant of the hair follicles and sebaceous glands, around, or even within, cancers of the skin in man.

For Borrel there was now no shadow of doubt whatever; to him the intervention of a parasite was obvious, though he did not assign it a direct role in causation. Cancer being due to a virus, an opinion that Borrel never relinquished, the parasite must act merely as its inoculator. Chance bearer of a carcinogenic virus, threading its way through the tissues, it infects in its progress whatever cells happen to lie in its path.

This brilliant hypothesis had the misfortune to be announced at a time when it still lacked any scientific foundation and the idea of a carcinogenic virus seemed the purest fantasy, for although it was supported by an observation or two here and there these could easily be explained away as coincidences; no experimental demonstration had yet been provided. Then, too, the role of Demodex in cancer of the skin seemed more than problematical, for the parasite occurred with equal frequency in cancers and in normal skin.

Discredited from the first by this medley of findings, true enough, to be sure, but unverified, and by more than questionable inferences, the parasitic hypothesis had little to commend it. It fell into complete oblivion, therefore, from which it could be rescued only by such dramatic testimony as that of Fibiger.

His experiments are among the most brilliant in all the domain of cancer research, and constitute a scientific odyssey that cannot be too often retold. Busy with an investigation of tuberculosis, he had occasion one day to autopsy three rats that had been inoculated with the bacillus of this disease. The animals, which had been kept in one cage and had all died on the same day, showed no sign of tuberculosis, but in the stomach of each there were large, tumor-like masses in the cardiac end, or forestomach, as it is often called. The presence of identical growths in three rats that had lived in such close contact suggested an infectious process of some sort, and the inquiry was accordingly turned in this direction. Bits of the tumors were inoculated into one group of rats, fed to a second, and a third lot was assigned to the cage that had housed the original three.

All these experiments were negative.

The fragments that had been preserved for microscopic examination confirmed the diagnosis of neoplasm. The tumors were vigorously proliferating papillomas of the ordinary, cauliflower type, only they contained numerous round or oval bodies that were sometimes bordered by traces of a horny cuticle. Although these structures resembled cross sections of a parasite, none of the authorities consulted could identify it, so Fibiger set about reconstructing it from serial sections, and had the good fortune to find a whole parasite that ran through 900 of these. It proved to be a small nematode worm, with tapering ends and about 1.5 centimeters, or something over half an inch, in length, but still wholly unfamiliar. It appeared to belong to an unknown variety, and inquiry among the various laboratories confirmed this impression for neither McCoy, who had autopsied about 100,000 rats, nor Borrel, who had examined about 8,000, had ever seen anything like it, and a search of the literature was no more helpful.

Meanwhile Fibiger continued his experiments. Eleven hundred rats were trapped in Copenhagen, and while an occasional nematode was found it was not the one in which he was interested and, more important still, no tumors were discovered. Puzzled by this failure, he then traced down the origin of his first three rats and learned that they had come from Dorpat; but the dealer, having retired from business, could no longer be found, so all hope of getting more animals from the same source had to be abandoned. The thread was broken, and anyone else would have given up.

But Fibiger was a man of uncommon mold. Obviously there was no longer any chance of finding his worm in rats, but parasites of its sort generally do not pass their entire life cycle in the same species, and as the adult nematode had been found in the stomach of a rat there was every probability that its larval form would be found in another species, that served as an intermediate host. But what species?

Exhaustive search of the literature at last uncovered the clue. In an old periodical there was discovered a paper by Galeb describing a nematode, parasitic in the stomach of the rat, that the author identified with a thread worm reported in 1824 by Deslongchamps. Its larval form developed in the fat body of the common European cockroach, *Blatta orientalis.* As neither of these papers mentioned a tumor Fibiger had no way of knowing whether this parasite was the same as his, but the possibility that the cockroach might be the intermediate host of his elusive nematode immediately suggested a new approach to his problem.

First, he must try to find out where rats and cockroaches lived together. "Nothing easier," came the reply. "In every old bakery in Copenhagen." In conformity with this answer rats and cockroaches innumerable were gathered, but both nematodes and tumors were sought in vain.

Five years had now gone by since the three tumor-bearing rats had been found, and the riddle presented by the discovery of parasites in their neoplasms was no nearer solution than ever. Fibiger was about to give up in despair when he heard of a sugar refinery in the suburbs of Copenhagen where rats and cockroaches abounded. The cockroaches obtained from this building were not *Blatta orientalis,* so common throughout Europe, but a different species, *Blatta americana,* that had reached Denmark on sugar cane from America.

The first three rats trapped in this refinery had the long-sought nematodes in their stomachs, mature forms with eggs in generous quantity! A grand raid then furnished 61 rats, of which 21 were normal and 40 infested with parasites containing eggs; and 9 of the infested rats had tumors, of which some were unquestionably carcinomas.

The problem was solved.

The carcinogenic worm, to which Fibiger gave the name *Gongylonema neoplasticum,* soon changed to *Spiroptera neoplastica,* lives in the stomach of the rat. Cockroaches, eating the rat's excrement, become infested with the eggs, which develop in their bodies as far as the larval stage. When a cockroach thus parasitized is devoured by a rat the larvae are set free in the animal's stomach and penetrate its walls, where they attain maturity.

That must be the life cycle of the nematode, though it still had to be proved. The really important thing to do, however, was to infest large numbers of rats and study the role of the worm in the production of tumors for that, after all, was the fundamental problem.

Well, at that very moment the providential sugar refinery went up in flames, and all the rats and cockroaches with it. Fortunately, however, Fibiger had kept some of each in his laboratory, and when he examined the insects in serial sections he found larvae, not in the fat body, where lived the larval form of Deslongchamps' thread worm, but in the muscles of the thorax and legs. By feeding these infested roaches he succeeded in parasitizing rats, and even mice, thus reproducing experimentally the life cycle that he had foreseen.

Of 102 rats thus infested 54 developed tumors of the stomach rather promptly, after the short latent period of 2 or 3 months. At autopsy this organ was found full of large outgrowths that involved most of the squamous epithelial lining of its esophageal portion, and microscopic examination showed them to be papillomas which, after the lapse of a certain time, underwent the malignant change and invaded one after another the layers of the stomach wall. Their malignant nature was further proved by the appearance of metastases, in the lymph nodes most frequently but sometimes in the lungs. As there were always large numbers of parasites in the gastric tumors, but none in the secondary growths, it was clear that the neoplasm, once started, did not require their presence for its continued proliferation.

Occasionally the worms were set free in the mouth and, penetrating the tongue, elicited tumors there also; hence to the 54 papillomas of the stomach produced in these experiments there must be added 6 of the tongue. It is a curious fact, however, that the squamous epithelium of the esophagus, though identical with that of the forestomach and often invaded by Spiroptera, never gave rise to a neoplasm.

Mice proved much more resistant than rats to the carcinogenic action of the nematode, for of 300 infested only 3 developed tumors.

When its results were published, in 1914, this brilliant investigation aroused universal admiration, but the ensuing discussion brought three different interpretations of the connection between parasite and neoplasm.

Adherents of the irritation hypothesis denied to the Spiroptera any specific carcinogenic influence, preferring to believe that its action is never direct and that it merely sets up a chronic irritation that leads in the end to cancer.

Fibiger himself thought that the worm acts in a specific manner, by excreting toxic substances that stimulate epithelial growth.

Borrel never receded from the position that he had taken from the first. For him, neither the Spiroptera nor any other parasite can provoke a malignant tumor unless contaminated with a carcinogenic virus. Then, as it penetrates the epithelium, it infects the cells, succeeding where the laboratory fails because its manipulations are so infinitely more delicate than those of the investigator's inoculating needle. Borrel found support for his belief in the capricious accomplishments of parasites, which do or do not evoke cancer, he thought, according to whether virus is or is not present, and he predicted that some experiments would have a negative outcome just because it happened to be absent.

Needless to say, it was Borrel's explanation that was adjudged the least probable, and most investigators did not even take the trouble to discuss it.

The story of Spiroptera cancer is not yet complete. Fibiger gained the highest rewards to which a scientific man may aspire but, himself falling victim to cancer of the stomach, soon had to relinquish his work. Others, however, took it up where he had dropped it. Bonne reported 1 successful result in 7 infested rats, Brumpt another among 300, Yokogawa 7 among 44 parasitized gray Norway rats, and Nishimura 8 among 91 white rats, but it became increasingly evident that even though the nematode does produce tumors no one could elicit them so regularly as Fibiger. Furthermore, negative observations began to accumulate. Among thousands of infested rats examined by Seurat, Yokogawa, Falko, Fielding, and Tubangui, not one had tumors in its stomach. Brumpt, finally, infested 55 piebald rats, all of which remained free of neoplasms, but this experiment was on too small a scale to permit definite conclusions.

A revision of the whole question was obviously imperative, and Passey, Leese, and Knox applied themselves to the task. They succeeded in obtaining rats infested with Spiroptera and in reëstablishing the life cycle as Fibiger had done, but to their amazement none of their parasitized rats developed papillomas. With indefatigable patience they began all over again. They made experiment after experiment, they took pains to get from Fibiger's laboratory all the details concerning diet and any other factors that might have some bearing on the result, they repeated everything exactly as Fibiger had done it, and still the outcome was negative. After years of work these English investigators were unable to point to one single Spiroptera neoplasm.

In the meantime the absence of certain vitamins had been suggested as a cause of tumors. Now Fibiger had fed his rats on white bread and water, a diet notably poor in vitamins and wholly lacking in vitamin A, and it was probably this that in 1926 led the Japanese investigator Fujimaki to see whether such a deficiency alone would be sufficient to produce gastric tumors. The result of his experiments seemed fully to justify his suspicion, for he obtained a most impressive crop of papillomas, which were identical in many ways with those of Fibiger; later, however, in 1931, he ascribed them to fatty acids rather than to vitamin A deprivation.

Cramer was unable to confirm Fujimaki's earlier statement, for old stock rats that had been maintained on a full ration were also found to have papillomas of the stomach. His experiments have their counterpart in the equally curious findings described by Pappenheimer and Larrimore. In rats kept on a rachitogenic diet, a regimen deficient in vitamin D, they discovered papillomas of the stomach; but these occurred also when vitamin D, in the form of cod-liver oil, was added to the food.

Thus gastric tumors have been seen in rats maintained on variously deficient diets, and sometimes even in those adequately nourished, and all in the absence of parasites. It has been impossible so far to identify the cause of these growths, but some alimentary influence is suspected. In such a case the parasite would have to be content with the role of any banal irritant in determining the site of a neoplasm.

Such was the situation in 1936, when Cramer repeated his experiment. His final conclusion was that while unbalanced diets, and especially those deficient in vitamin A, may play a contributory part in the etiology of gastric papillomatosis, they are not the chief determining factor, for the lesions do not always appear on such a regime. The question is complex, and during the past few years it has stimulated a whole series of experiments, among which may be mentioned those of Fridericia, Gudjonsson, Vimtrup, and J. and S. Clemmesen, of Fibiger's laboratory, and of Brunschwig and Rasmussen, yet the problem has not been solved. In a few words, papillary outgrowths may be inaugurated on any sort of deficient regimen, particularly those poor in proteins and vitamin A, but there is no regularity in their occurrence and, more baffling still, they sometimes arise in rats that enjoy a full diet.

No, the problem has not been solved. It has had a strange career, and evidently conceals one or more entirely unsuspected factors. Every time that it has seemed on the eve of solution the control experiments have upset everything. Every time that the responsible factor has seemed to be in sight further investigation has shown it to be accessory at the most.

One cannot help thinking of Borrel, of Borrel who predicted all this. Could not one of these unrecognized factors be a virus? The question, it must be confessed, becomes more and more justifiable though further than this, unhappily, it is impossible to go at the moment. It would be foolhardy to assert the existence of a virus without conclusive experimental proof of its presence, but it is to be hoped that the next investigator to encounter papillomas of the rat's stomach will not fail to consider the possibility and to make all the appropriate tests.

Among other experiments on the relation of parasites to tumors must be mentioned the work of Bullock and Curtis on the sarcoma of the rat's liver that follows infestation with *Cysticercus fasciolaris.* Borrel, who first observed it, had already attempted artificial infestation but had to interrupt his work for lack of means. The Americans resumed it with success.

The adult form of this parasite, *Taenia crassicollis,* lives in the intestine of the cat. Its eggs, passed with the feces, are eaten by rats, enter the walls of their digestive tracts, penetrate the vessels, and so are carried to the liver where they develop the larval form and become encysted. The cycle is completed when an infested rat is eaten by a cat, in whose intestinal tract the larvae mature and become tapeworms.

Bullock and Curtis parasitized rats by feeding them watery emulsions of cat feces containing 10 to 60 eggs. In a first series of experiments 1,165 were thus infested, but the first 600, killed and examined 5 months later, had no tumors. The time had been too short, for sarcomas were found in 29 per cent of those killed after a longer interval. They arose from 8 to 15 months after infestation, in the connective tissue walls of the cysts enclosing the larvae, and in structure were spindle or polymorphous cell sarcomas, with an occasional chondrosarcoma. The determining role of the parasite in their production was proved by implanting young cysts in the subcutaneous tissue, where they elicited sarcomas just as they do in the liver.

In these experiments there appeared once more the fact that Borrel had so often and so strongly emphasized; the tumors developed in some of the parasitized animals only, not in all. In an attempt to explain this Curtis, Dunning, and Bullock repeated the experiment on thousands of animals and reported 3,285 sarcomas in 26,172 infested rats that had survived more than 8 months, but the percentage of sarcomas was hardly any higher than before. Unlike Borrel, they referred the large number of negative results to constitutional and hereditary factors, and to mutation.

More recently Bonne and Sandground have described another type of parasitic tumor that appeared at autopsy in the stomach of the Javanese monkey *Macacus mordax,* more commonly known as

Macacus cynomolgus, as a polypoid neoplasm containing a number of nematode worms. A systematic inquiry was thereupon instituted that led to the discovery of 6 similar growths among 68 monkeys selected at random and killed for examination. The worms, identified as *Nochtia nochti,* a genus of the suborder *Strongyloidea,* were never seen superficially but could easily be stimulated to emerge from the tumors in which they live by immersing the empty stomach in a warm bath of physiological saline solution.

The growths induced by these nematodes were cauliflower-like masses, situated near the pylorus, and microscopic examination showed them to be adenomas with a definite tendency to invade the stomach wall; in one instance a blood vessel had been attacked, but no metastases were found.

Though the life cycle of this parasite has not yet been worked out, Bonne and Sandground think that some part of it may be passed outside the body of the monkey, and that infestation occurs by way of the mouth. When their article appeared two monkeys had been experimentally parasitized. Under general anesthesia the stomach was opened, and after the investigators had assured themselves that the organ was entirely normal adult worms were introduced into it. Two and three months later typical growths, containing the parasites, were found.

The examples given are by no means the only parasites that are capable of giving rise to neoplasms. With no idea of complete enumeration we may mention, in man, *Distoma hepaticum* (*Fasciola hepatica*), the common liver fluke of herbivorous animals, which sometimes elicits tumors of the bile passages; *Schistosoma mansoni* and *Schistosoma japonicum* (the Asiatic blood fluke), which may induce carcinoma of the intestine or liver; and *Onchocerca volvulus,* which incites the fibromatous growths studied by R. P. Strong. In the sheep there is *Strongylus filaria,* which causes "sheep cough," a disease of the lungs that is sometimes associated with cancer; and finally, in the rat, *Hepaticola gastrica,* a parasite that produces a carcinoma of the stomach differing from Spiroptera cancer in its combination with sarcoma.

The conclusion to be drawn from the work described in this section is that parasites, by their presence, may be a cause of neoplasia, but that the problem is not quite so easy as at first sight it appears to be, for the effect is far from constant. Fibiger's Spiroptera elicited tumors in 54 per cent of infested rats, the highest proportion yet attained; generally the number is much smaller and there can be little doubt that some factor is required over and above the mere presence of a parasite. For Borrel this was a carcinogenic virus, for Curtis, Dunning, and Bullock constitutional and hereditary influences and mutation, for others diet. We shall see in the following pages what to make of all these different explanations.

HEREDITARY FACTORS IN CANCER

A VISIT to the laboratory of a geneticist is always a profoundly moving experience. Nowhere else is there to be had such a vivid sensation of penetrating to the very heart of nature, for here can be seen in operation all the mysterious influences upon which our destiny depends: health and disease, physical and mental equilibrium, traits of character no less than external appearance, in short the whole gamut of our being. And man, learning little by little to unravel the laws that determine all these things, learns at the same time to mold the organism according to his will.

The geneticist moves among his animals as though endowed with a spark of divinity that permits him to fix the course of their lives even before they are born. He shows us strains bred for longevity, since by judicious matings continued through many generations he has eliminated any weaknesses upon which disease might lay hold and so is able to guarantee a life span of more than ordinary length.

Then he shows us other strains that are resistant to cancer. The disease can be produced in them artificially, of course, with powerful carcinogenic agents like the X rays or suitable chemical compounds, but left to themselves they will never have it; it has vanished from their strain. The immunity to spontaneous cancer that Ehrlich strove so vainly to realize, by inducing resistance against a variety of transplantable tumors, is achieved by genetics through the natural process of selection.

Before we leave we are shown strains of which every member will die of cancer; it is indissolubly linked to their fate. Even its very site determined, the disease will appear at a predestined time as though it were a natural event and as inevitably as puberty or the menopause.

Such are the facts. We shall see next how they have been obtained, what is their application to cancer in man, and what their significance for the cancer problem in general.

It is a mere platitude to say that there is often a resemblance among members of the same family, and it is almost as well known that certain traits may be present in grandparents and their grandchildren without having appeared in the parents. This ability of hereditary characteristics to skip one generation, or even several, puzzled naturalists for many years, and only toward the middle of the past century was an explanation forthcoming. Naudin announced it as a hypothesis and Gregor Mendel, an Austrian monk, showed it to be true by irrefutable experiments, for he it was who established the laws by which heredity can be charted, as it were, and upon which all modern genetics rests.

Mendel obtained his results by employing two procedures that were ingenious novelties at the time but, like all great things, simple at bottom.

All preceding attempts to solve the riddles of heredity had failed because investigators tried to envisage at once all the characters that they could find in their experimental material. Such was the complexity, therefore, that even the most salient facts were masked and so escaped discovery. Mendel reduced the problem to its simplest terms by taking into account only one characteristic at a time. He crossed plants belonging to the same species, peas, for example, but bearing blossoms of different colors, studied carefully this first hybrid generation, then crossed these hybrid plants among themselves, and so on, paying attention only to blossom color and closing his eyes to leaves, stems, and seeds. Not until he had established the law of hybridization for single characters did he venture to attack the problem of their combinations.

His second innovation was to employ the numerical, or statistical, method. By recording scrupulously the number of plants in each generation that presented such and such a character he discovered that there is always a definite proportion between the numbers of individuals of one type and those of the other, thus casting an entirely new light on the conceptions of heredity then current.

In examining this, the first of Mendel's two laws, for our present purpose the more interesting, we shall take as examples not plants, but animals, the Andalusian fowl and the mouse.

Crossing a black Andalusian cock with a white hen, or vice versa, results in hybrids that appear to resemble neither one of the parents; their plumage looks blue. But a stable variety has not been created, for actually the gametes, that is the ova and spermatozoa, of these birds contain a mixture in equal parts of the factors capable of producing black or white, and it is the simultaneous presence of these two factors that determines the blue appearance of the feathers.

That this is so can be shown by crossing these hybrids among themselves. The black-white gametes will interchange their factors with those of other gametes, also black-white, to form new pairs. Four combinations are possible: black-black, white-white, black-white, or white-black, the two latter being identical from a practical point of view. Obviously the chickens with similar gametes (*homozygotes*), black-black or white-white, will be black or white respectively, whereas those with mixed gametes (*heterozygotes*), black-white or white-black, will be blue.

This is what takes place: the crossing of hybrids among themselves leads to a separation, or *segregation*, of the mixed factors and there will appear black, white, and blue descendants in the proportion 1:1:2, which is exactly what the hypothesis demands. In succeeding generations the process is repeated indefinitely; whites crossed together have white offspring; the blacks have black; and the blue hybrids, crossed among themselves, always have 25 per cent of white, 25 per cent of black, and 50 per cent of blue hybrid descendants.

And now for our second example, the crossing of a gray with a white mouse. The offspring of the first generation will be gray hybrids, and their gametes, like those in the preceding example, will be mixed, gray-white; but here the heterozygote character will not appear in their coats because one of the factors, the gray, is *dominant*. The white factor, which is suppressed, is called the *recessive*.

These gray hybrids are a variety no more stable than the blue hybrid Andalusian chickens, and when they are crossed among themselves the result will be 25 per cent pure gray, homozygous, mice; 25 per cent white, homozygous, mice; and 50 per cent gray hybrid, or heterozygous, mice. The first two varieties are stable, but members of the third group, when crossed among themselves, will always produce the same proportion of whites, pure grays, and hybrid grays.

A hybrid can never be recognized by ordinary examination. A heterozygous gray mouse cannot be distinguished from a homozygous gray mouse, and when mated even for many generations gray hybrids and pure grays together will always produce gray mice. But the recessive character will appear as soon as two hybrids are crossed, and 25 per cent of their descendants will be white.

Thus a hereditary character, if it be recessive, may lie concealed for many generations; but when two recessives meet in procreation the character appears once more in the offspring.

The ground having been cleared, we may return to the cancer problem.

Before any serious work on the inheritance of cancer could be started it had to be known whether or not neoplasia really does depend on a character that is subject to the laws of heredity. Preliminary inquiries in several mouse colonies suggested that it does, for J. A. Murray, Lathrop and Loeb, Tyzzer, and others had observed the appearance of tumors in great number among mice of cancerous ancestry that had long been bred among themselves, and the rarity of neoplasms in those of noncancerous ancestry similarly interbred. But the establishment of pure "cancer" or "noncancer" strains is no easy matter. In genetic studies on coat color in mice, or blossom color in plants, the strains with which to work are available from the first; a few crosses between animals or plants of the same nature and the investigator knows whether the character in which he is interested is transmitted or not, whether it is dominant or recessive. With cancer it is not so. The necessary strains must first be developed.

Here was revealed the infinite patience of Maud Slye. One day, still only a girl, she burst into the pathological laboratory of H. Gideon Wells, in Chicago, exclaiming that she simply must study the heredity of cancer and would need some mice and a corner of his laboratory. Well, the few mice became a thousand, then ten thousand, then hundreds of thousands, and the modest corner to which she had been assigned became an institute where they were housed under the most perfect conditions, pedigreed, selectively bred, observed throughout their lives, and at last autopsied with scrupulous care.

To understand the infinite pains required in founding a line that is genetically pure with respect to a given character it must be recalled that every character of an individual is represented in the chromosomes of his sex cells by a minute corpuscle called a *gene*. In man there are 48 chromosomes, and in every chromosome are aligned thousands of genes. Before full maturation of ova and spermatozoa half their chromosomes are eliminated, a process that removes at random some genes derived from the male and some from the female parent. At the moment of fecundation 2 sex cells fuse to form 1, the fertilized ovum, which thus acquires the complete number of chromosomes.

Obviously, then, fertilization accomplished through the hazards of nature between genetically different partners will result in so many different combinations that among millions of individuals no two will be alike. But nature's gamble may be modified experimentally, directed, in a way, by selecting consanguine mates and continuing to breed in this way for generation after generation.

According to the law of probability, several among the issue of a breeding pair will possess the same character, eye or coat color, say, or, in insects, wing shape, and if a brother and sister thus equipped be crossed the character in question will emerge in a certain number of their descendants. Systematic repetition of the process among these will eventually produce a strain all members of which possess it. In respect to this character the strain is now genetically pure.

This is the method that was followed in the Chicago laboratory to establish pure cancer and noncancer strains, but the problem was much more difficult than any ordinary experiment in heredity. For if animals are to be selected for a character like coat color it will very soon be known in which descendants it has appeared, and those in which it has not can be promptly discarded, since there is no need of crossing them further. It is quite different with cancer, a disease that does not assert itself until more or less advanced age. Here it is essential to keep all the animals, make all the crosses, and hold all the issue for observation until the death of the parents from natural causes. Not until then, after both parents have been autopsied, can the fate of their descendants be settled and only those retained for further breeding whose parents had cancer.

This will give some idea of the enormous amount of patient and methodical work demanded by such an inquiry. Every possible measure must be taken to prevent early death from disease, for if an animal were to die prematurely all the descendants would be useless since there would be no way of determining whether or not it would have developed a tumor had it lived on into the cancer age. Thus the mice must be housed under ideal sanitary conditions and constantly guarded against early death from disease or accident. Or again, one single error in a crossing may ruin several years' work; yet in spite of all these difficulties mouse strains were developed in which cancer seized almost all the members, and others that were resistant to the disease.

Cancer strains naturally include lines whose members are susceptible to that most common variety of mouse cancer, carcinoma of the mammary gland, but there are others in addition that are prone to pulmonary carcinoma, carcinoma of the liver, carcinoma of the thyroid, and sarcoma of the upper jaw. The sarcoma is especially interesting, for it is associated with a dental anomaly, deviation of an upper incisor. The corresponding incisor in the lower jaw, not being worn away as it normally would be by friction against its upper companion, grows inordinately long, constantly wounds the upper gum, and it is just at this point that the sarcoma always appears. Early extraction of the lower tooth prevents the neoplasm from developing.

These observations, and many others made by Maud Slye in the course of her long experience, are impressive, for in performing something like 200,000 autopsies on mice she has seen virtually all the tumors encountered in the human subject.

But the founding of pure strains was, after all, only a preliminary. The results, it is true, have been of the highest importance since they have proved beyond any doubt that certain cancers are associated with hereditary factors, but it still remained to discover how these factors would be transmitted when a mouse of a cancer strain was crossed with one from another cancer strain, or with one from a noncancer strain.

The results at first seemed unequivocal. Crossing an animal from a cancer strain with one from a noncancer strain gave a generation of hybrids that were exempt from cancer. In the second generation, however, it appeared in a certain number, and arose, too, in mice obtained by crossing the hybrids that did not develop it. The tendency to develop cancer seemed to be transmitted according to mendelian laws, and appeared to be recessive, whereas resistance behaved as a dominant. In brief, cancer acted as does albinism in the crossing of gray and white mice.

These experiments, which attracted considerable attention, were repeated on all sides by geneticists, Little, Lynch, L. C. Strong, MacDowell and Richter, and Dobrovolskaïa-Zavadskaïa among them, and on the whole the first part of the work was confirmed. Cancer strains have been established in many laboratories and have already furnished the basis for truly impressive experiments. Mice in which cancer may be expected to appear on a certain fixed date, so to speak, would be an ideal material in which to study the changes preceding it, but unfortunately the small size of these animals has been an obstacle, for most of the changes are of a physicochemical or humoral order and it is difficult to get sufficient material. Accordingly the field has recently been extended to include the rabbit and results of great interest have been obtained, particularly with mammary cancer, by Greene.

Two main objections have been raised against these pure cancer and noncancer strains.

First, a malignant tumor appears from time to time in a "noncancer" strain. This, however, shows only that hereditary transmission does not apply to every single neoplasm. As has been explained in a preceding paragraph, tumors can be elicited with X rays or carcinogenic chemical compounds even in a noncancer strain, but this is no reason for denying any and all hereditary influence. On a willing subject a skillful surgeon could easily make a harelip. It would be an acquired harelip, but would it justify an assertion that the congenital nature of harelip had not been substantiated? The factors responsible for cancer are many, and heredity is one of them. If others also are operative this does not warrant the elimination of heredity in cases where it is manifestly in play.

Secondly, much has been made of the fact that some animals belonging to "cancer" strains never develop cancer. In order to answer this objection we must recall the fundamental distinction between a hereditary *factor* and a hereditary *character*. A character is the expression of a factor, and just as the latent photographic image must be developed to make it visible, so must there be a "revelatory condition" of some sort if a hereditary factor is to be realized. In other words, a hereditary factor may exist with no outward sign of its presence, as the following illustration well shows. In a variety of corn with red kernels this color depends upon a hereditary factor, but red does not appear unless the plant is exposed to the sun; ears protected from the light stay yellow, even though the red factor is there.

Cancer itself, too, furnishes some striking examples of this. Mammary carcinoma in the mouse is associated with a hereditary factor, but it is evident that follicular hormone is required in addition, for removal of the ovaries a day or so after birth prevents the appearance of cancer in later life, as Leo Loeb has shown. Conversely, the injection of follicular hormone will elicit mammary carcinoma in male mice, which ordinarily never have it even though they belong to cancer strains. Finally, there is that striking example, just referred to, of the relation between a dental malformation and sarcoma of the jaw. The factor for the neoplasm requires injury if it is to be evinced, since preventing the trauma prevents the sarcoma, even though its factor is there.

Thus the factor for cancer may be present but not manifest. Follicular hormone for mammary cancer of the mouse, and traumatism for this sarcoma, are the revelatory conditions that have been recognized, but surely there are many others of which we are still wholly ignorant. If cancer does not always arise, then, in every single mouse of a cancer strain, the presence of a hereditary factor is by no means precluded thereby.

We come now to Maud Slye's second series of experiments, on the way in which the cancer factor is transmitted.

There have been many objections to her conclusion that cancer is recessive and resistance dominant, and both Marsh and Lynch, for example, maintain that mammary carcinoma in the mouse depends on a dominant factor. It should be explained, however, that dominance today has not the absolute value formerly attributed to it; indeed, it may be incomplete or even absent.

In any case the general impression seems to be that cancer in man is a recessive rather than a dominant character. On the one hand, it attacks persons whose ancestors have escaped it and, on the other, descendants of those who have had cancer may never get the disease. This would be inexplicable if the factor for cancer were dominant.

In this connection one of Maud Slye's experiments is enlightening. If cancer is recessive hybrids will not develop it. Now while investigating a strain of mice subject to cancer of the thyroid gland she made many generations of crosses between hybrids and mice that had not been selectively bred for this type of neoplasm without ever once seeing a single cancer of the thyroid. Yet when hybrids were crossed among themselves the tumor regularly appeared. Such an experiment is convincing to a degree, but it must be confessed that the facts do not always emerge so clearly. On the contrary, the more the experiments are multiplied the more complicated, not to say obscure, does the situation become, and at present it seems almost certain that cancer depends not on one but on several mendelian factors. Even Maud Slye herself had to recognize at least two: one for *localization*, and one for *malignancy* in every variety of neoplasm (carcinoma, sarcoma, leukemia, and so on).

Once the existence of multiple factors was admitted the problem became more than complex, for according to the second law of Mendel these are transmitted independently of one another and some may be recessive and others dominant. Moreover, it becomes increasingly evident from the investigations of Little, W. S. Murray, Cloudman, and others that the conditions for hereditary transmission may be different for different varieties of tumors, and the confusion that has resulted has never been more concisely put than in Warthin's little jest: The heredity of cancer seems to be dominant in some cases, recessive in others, while in the remainder it is a matter of heads or tails.

Finally, the work of the past few years has confirmed an idea, held now for some time by certain geneticists like Little, that the heredity of cancer may not depend upon chromosomal factors alone but upon something quite different. Today it is known how this something is transmitted; it is by the "milk influence" of Bittner, to which we shall return in a subsequent chapter.

The idea overturns the classical theories of heredity, and its application to cancer will exert effects that cannot possibly be foreseen at the present time. Certainly it goes far beyond the first simple concept of Maud Slye, and we may conclude our discussion by saying that the intervention of hereditary factors in the genesis of certain neoplasms has been proved beyond any doubt, but that the way in which they are transmitted is so much a matter of dispute that years of investigation will be required to bring order out of chaos.

And now comes the question: How do all these facts apply to cancer in the human subject?

The facile but unscientific procedure of condemning them all out of hand because they were gathered by experimenting on the mouse is wholly deplorable. Heredity is one of the most general concepts in the entire domain of biology and there is every chance that laws applicable to mouse or rabbit will hold good for man himself, particularly in the case of malignant tumors, which are so similar no matter in what species they arise. Furthermore, the hereditary transmission of susceptibility in man is supported by direct and irrefutable proof.

As a first example may be mentioned those neoplasms that often attack monochorial twins in identical manner, involving not only the same organ but the same part of this organ, and appearing at the same age. Then, too, there are similar observations on brothers and sisters that were not twins. No doubt there should be brought up here those famous twins who, according to McFarland and Meade, each lost a left leg in battle during the Civil War, but this is more a pleasantry than a serious objection for concordant tumors in twins are certainly more common than identical injuries.

Secondly, some tumors such as glioma of the retina, the neurofibromas of Recklinghausen's disease, and polyps of the large intestine are hereditary beyond any doubt.

In the third place, there are certain statistical findings, which, however, are to be accepted only with caution. Immediately there arises the moot question of "cancer families." Though the classic examples are the not very convincing Bonaparte family, and the Broca family, under observation for seven generations with an extraordinary number of cancer deaths, far better ones are available. There are, for instance, the two families recorded by Paulsen. In the first the father, mother, and 6 children died of cancer of the stomach; the only member to escape the disease was lost in an accident at the age of 28 years. In the second family the mother and 6 children succumbed to cancer of the stomach; according to his death certificate the father died of intestinal obstruction, but it is almost certain that he, too, had cancer of the stomach.

In a family studied by Warthin there were 175 individuals in 4 generations, of whom 41 died of cancer. The neoplasms showed a distinct predilection for the gastrointestinal tract (26 cases) and the body of the uterus (15 cases).

Such facts as these seem really impressive, but care must be taken not to attribute to "cancer families" more importance than they deserve. In most instances the explanation given for "cancer houses" and "cancer cages" will apply; in a disease as common as cancer there will inevitably be, just by chance, an accumulation of cases in some families and a total absence in others, quite apart from any question of heredity.

To guard against error a more substantial foundation has been sought in statistics on the frequency of cancer among the ancestors of persons with or without the disease. Yet even this method conceals many sources of error. The outcome is deeply influenced by subjective factors, for as the causes of death in the ascendants are not always accurately known the investigator has nothing to go on but the symptoms described to him. His interpretation of these is colored by his faith in, or distrust of, the hereditary transmission of a susceptibility to cancer and, as might have been expected, the results of such inquiries show anywhere from 2 to 30 per cent of cancerous antecedents among cancer patients.

Again, though certain types of cancer are associated with hereditary tendencies it is almost certain that other types are not, and when statistics are gathered on a large scale, all cancers being included without discrimination, error can be almost guaranteed. To avoid it, Wassink, in Holland, and Waaler, in Norway, took into consideration only neoplasms at the same site. They found four varieties that clearly show a familial tendency: cancers of the breast, uterus, prostate, and stomach.

But the chief source of error in all these investigations is that the recessive cases escape discovery, because the only way of recognizing a recessive factor in a hybrid is the hybridization test, that is, crossing with another recessive. If the factor for malignant neoplasia is a recessive all statistics on the ancestry of cancer patients are shorn of significance. In the experiment with thyroid cancer, described in a preceding paragraph, as many negative generations as desired could be obtained merely by crossing hybrids with mice taken at random from nonselected stocks. For a statistician there would be no thyroid cancer in the family, yet by crossing hybrids among themselves the investigator could make cancer appear at will.

Though actual proof is no easy matter, there can be little doubt that heredity does play some part in the determination of neoplasms in the human subject. But how large a part?

There are few ideas so imperfectly understood as heredity, or that give rise to so much shaky reasoning, especially in its relation to cancer. He who accepts its intervention immediately identifies this with predestined liability to disaster, with a fate settled at the time of conception, with a mere passive waiting to see what will turn up next.

Nothing could be further from the truth.

It has repeatedly been emphasized that hereditary factors do not apply to all cancers. Many agents are known with which neoplasms can be elicited experimentally when and where we will, and in man there are tumors induced by external influences alone. All these can be easily forestalled, since their causes are known, a fact to which the prevention of industrial cancer is eloquent witness.

But even those new growths that depend upon hereditary factors may be influenced by prophylactic measures, and certainly will become even more amenable in the future. After all, it is not *cancer* that is transmitted but a *cancer factor*, and it has already been explained that a factor is not manifested invariably but only under certain conditions. Consider once more xeroderma pigmentosum. To a superficial observer this would seem to be a hereditary cancer, but what really is transmitted is not cancer at all but a sensitivity of the skin to sunlight. A person with such a skin would never have cancer if he passed his life in the depths of a cave.

The relationship of hormones to mammary cancer in mice is probably valid for man also. What is hereditarily transmitted is not cancer of the mamma, but an abnormal sensitivity of the mammary epithelium to follicular hormone, and when a way has been found to counteract the effect of the hormone, cancer of the breast will be a preventable disease.

A perfect example of this is a condition recently investigated by Wassink, of Amsterdam, and Ahlbohm, of Stockholm. In 1936 they showed that cancer of the mouth, throat, and esophagus in women is often preceded by a form of anemia in which the secretion of gastric juice is diminished or absent. It may persist from youth, and is accompanied by a group of other manifestations known collectively for years as the Plummer-Vinson syndrome. There is an early loss of the teeth, the nails are thin, soft, and concave ("spoon nails"), and the mucous membrane of the tongue, mouth, throat, and esophagus becomes atrophic, dry, pale, and tends to fissure. The condition can be cured easily by the administration of iron and hydrochloric acid, and its cure prevents the cancer in which so often it otherwise terminates.

An analogous situation undoubtedly exists in the case of most neoplasms that depend upon the intervention of a hereditary factor. Whether it be in the stomach, the uterus, or the prostate, cancer rarely appears as a bolt from the blue. Almost always it is preceded by nutritional disturbances in the epithelium that masquerade under various names but that are, after all, merely the expression of an abnormal reactivity to certain influences. This is the place to look, and it may very well be that the means of correction will turn out to be just as simple as the administration of iron and hydrochloric acid for the Plummer-Vinson syndrome. The future may be faced with high hope.

A realization that hereditary factors underlie some varieties of malignant growth by no means condemns to fatalism. Quite otherwise. The fact that they do exist should demand a general revision of all the clinical findings and a systematic search for revelatory conditions, but as these probably differ for each variety of neoplasm patient and intensive study of each case will be required. Every tumor must be forced to reveal the story of its life.

We are too much swayed by the notion that there is only one cause for neoplasia, and that when this has been discovered all cancers will be explained as if by magic. A grave mistake. Even though the final cause were identical, the conditions under which they appear are different for all types of new growth, and prevention cannot succeed until these circumstances are understood and controlled. Against heredity there is no appeal, but the revelatory conditions that set its factors in action can be conquered.

A concluding word to those who feel themselves menaced because of cancer in their families. What, they ask in their anxiety, are the chances that they, too, will be attacked? A geneticist working with pure strains of mice could make such a forecast for the descendants of a pair whose every hereditary character he had rigorously analyzed, but in man it is wholly impossible. Here, for obvious reasons, there are not, nor can there ever be, strains that are pure from a genetic point of view, so that even with precise knowledge of a person's antecedents prediction would be vain.

Another thing to be kept in mind is our almost total ignorance of the various revelatory conditions. In experiments on the mouse they do not appear at their full value because this little denizen of the laboratory lives under entirely artificial surroundings. Whole populations go through life in the same cages, always at the same temperature, always on the same standardized diet, with everything done to regulate their existence and guard them from accident and disease; in short, to guarantee as long a life as possible. But because this is so all individual reaction, all that distinguishes one mouse from another, is suppressed. Amidst these calm and even surroundings hereditary factors are revealed with a regularity that makes us forget the importance of all those other external influences capable under more natural circumstances of favoring or preventing their appearance.

With man it is not so.

Think for but a moment of how the lives of different people vary from day to day in diet, housing, intellectual or muscular work; in harmful influences such as infections, injuries, industrial diseases, alcohol, tobacco, and so on. All the external influences that have been reduced to a minimum in the mouse colony are free to exert their fullest effect on man, and the manifestation of his hereditary factors is profoundly modified in consequence.

Once more our monochorial twins provide us with a convincing illustration. Although they are descended from the same cell and therefore have identical genetic constitutions, to expect that if one developed a neoplasm the other would invariably have a concordant neoplasm, that is, a similar growth at the same or a different site, would be to expect too much. All tumors are not dependent upon hereditary factors. As a matter of fact, concordance was found by Versluys in hardly more than 30 per cent of his cases; the other 70 per cent had discordant neoplasms, a tumor in one twin and not in the other, or different types at different sites. This hardly meets anticipation, to be sure, but it shows the great importance of external influences that have no connection whatsoever with heredity.

For him who walks in the valley of the shadow this should be a consoling thought. Even were he certain, from a genetic point of view, to die of cancer the truth is that he has a 70 per cent chance of escaping and ending his days in some other manner.

CARCINOGENIC CHEMICAL COMPOUNDS

ENGLAND has always been a land of chimneys, where the open fire, with its bed of wood or coal, enjoys a favor that is thoroughly justified by the cold and damp of the long winter months.

But chimneys have to be cleaned periodically of the thick, sooty layer that collects on their walls. This toilsome and dangerous job used to fall to the lot of 5- or 10-year-old boys, who alone could crawl through the intricate flues, and these little unfortunates, these "climbing boys," as they were called, often fell victim in later life to a remorseless disease that began as an ulceration of the scrotum. Known under the name of "chimney sweeper's disease," it made its appearance at the age of 20 or 25 and invariably caused death from cachexia, or from hemorrhage if the ulceration involved the walls of the blood vessels. Percivall Pott published a careful description of the malady in 1775, identified it as cancer, and thus won the distinction of having recorded the first industrial carcinoma.

The intricate old chimneys have long been gone and the little sweeps with them, but those who met soot in other trades continued to have cancer of the skin until cleanliness and other modern prophylactic methods combined to make it a rarity. When it does appear it arises after a latent period of 10 to 15 years, as in the case of the sweeps, and is inevitable if the exposure has been sufficiently prolonged. Even those who have changed their occupations in the meantime and have not touched soot for years may be attacked.

It has been said that chimney sweep's cancer occurred in and about the scrotum because the rubbing of the trousers ground particles of soot into the skin; but the rich supply of sebaceous glands in this region may have been a contributing factor, for the deleterious agent may have been dissolved in their fatty secretion and thus more easily absorbed.

In addition to its carbon the material that collects in chimneys contains the distillation products of coal and wood, all of which together make up tar. It is this latter mixture that causes the trouble, for cancer appears wherever it is handled, as among those who manufacture tarred paper or cloth, briquettes, and so forth. In all such instances the neoplasms involve the arms and forearms, those regions most exposed to the tar; but in shops where particles of tar or pitch may be suspended in the air as dust the scrotum is just as apt to be attacked. Though long contact is requisite, as has already been explained, there have been exceptional cases in which cancer has made its appearance suddenly, after a burn from boiling tar.

A second group of substances responsible for industrial cancer comprises the distillation products of petroleum. Experiment has proved that it is those of high boiling point such as lubricating oil, fuel oil, and asphalt, and also the residue, pitch, that are most deleterious.

Lubricating oil causes cotton spinner's cancer, a special variety of occupational carcinoma seen above all in England. The operators work at their machines in the hot and humid atmosphere that must be maintained in the mills, wearing very light clothing that soon becomes soaked with oil thrown from the spinning-mules, and here again the scrotum most commonly suffers.

All the other distillation products of coal and petroleum mentioned above exact equally every one its own toll in the industries concerned.

Of these highly inimical mixtures man himself was the first victim, as he was of the X rays, long before the production of cancer in animals by these agents had been thought of. There must be a latent period in cancer research just as truly as there is in carcinogenesis, for Percivall Pott's article was dated 1775 and it was about 140 years before tar was subjected to adequate experimental examination.

The Tar Tumor

When the work of Yamagiwa and Itchikawa on the initiation of carcinoma with tar was first published, between 1918 and 1921, it aroused various reactions.

Some said that the result was only to have been expected, and was merely a confirmation of clinical facts that had been known for years. As for any consequences that might flow from the discovery, extreme skepticism seemed the only attitude worthy of a cautious man, for how could tar cancer in animals possibly yield any information that had not already been furnished by tar cancer in the human subject?

Others, and it is pleasant to remember that these were in the majority, greatly admired the work of the Japanese investigators, which they recognized immediately as fraught with significance. Here at last was the long-sought and ardently desired means of eliciting cancer at any chosen site by a method so simple that anyone could employ it, and they looked forward to a whole series of interesting experiments on the early phases of carcinogenesis, on the reactions of the body to the gradual evolution of the malady, on many problems, in brief, that could not be approached by the older methods.

The outcome has largely justified all these hopes.

But first let us pay our respects to the doubters. It is always easy after the event to say that such and such an experimental verification was to have been expected. Clinical observation suggested that tar is carcinogenic, yes, but this was not actually known. It had to be proved, for in the biological sciences one fact demonstrated is worth a hundred suppositions, and it was especially necessary that the question be settled because previous investigators had applied tar in vain. As far back as 1889 Hanau had painted rats with it in the hope of eliciting cancer, and in 1894 Cazin made a similar experiment on dogs. Much later, in 1913, Haga rubbed pitch into the ears and scrotum in rabbits, and at about the same time Bayon injected tar into the rabbit's ear. All these attempts miscarried.

Why, then, were the Japanese authors successful?

Because they had on their side the two conditions necessary to accomplish an end in any experimental research; patience, and good luck. They suspected that all the previous failures had been due to premature abandonment of the work, and so began their effort with the resolve to continue applying tar for as long as might be requisite, even years if necessary, and until the death of the animals. That was the whole secret of their method. Nevertheless, they did have the good fortune to choose an animal in which cancer can be easily evoked, for if they had selected the guinea pig or the dog nature would have triumphed even over Japanese tenacity. The attempt would have failed with those of their predecessors.

The technic employed by Yamagiwa and Itchikawa could not have been simpler. They merely applied tar two or three times a week to the internal surface of the rabbit's ear, a site at which no spontaneous tumor had ever been observed in this species. Thus in case a neoplasm did arise during the experiment there would be virtually no chance at all that it was spontaneous in origin.

After two or three months had passed by warty outgrowths covered with thickened, horny epithelium began to appear in the painted area, and increased considerably in size during the months following. Some of these papillomas, composed principally of keratin, projected further and further from the skin surface to become cutaneous horns, whereas others were broad and flat from the first. Eventually the latter ulcerated, the cutaneous horns broke off leaving other ulcers, and when the ulcerative lesions thickened and hardened at the base and became fixed on the underlying tissues it was a sign that the malignant change had set in. The tumors continued to grow, invaded the surrounding healthy tissues, destroyed the cartilage of the ear, and sometimes metastasized to the regional lymph nodes.

The experiment was soon repeated in mice by Tsutsui, who found them even more susceptible than the rabbit, for the growths arose earlier and more frequently; with suitable technic, indeed, he was able to induce them in 90 to 100 per cent of his animals. Ever since then the mouse has been the animal of choice, not only for tar but for most other carcinogenic agents as well. The same simple method is employed. A little of the substance under investigation is applied twice or thrice weekly to the nape of the neck, an area chosen because it is more or less out of reach of the paws. Thus the animal, in scratching, cannot transfer the carcinogen to other parts of the body and so cause the appearance of neoplasms at remote sites that might complicate the experiment.

Tar has been tried in species other than the rabbit and the mouse, but generally with slight success. In the rat the rare tumors that emerge require two or three years for their inception. In the dog the outcome is sporadic and inconstant, some investigators having recorded melanomas whereas the efforts of others have gone unrewarded, even after protracted application. In the guinea pig every attempt has failed.

Thus there is a definite species sensitivity, but even in susceptible animals only certain tissues capitulate. The epithelium of the skin is responsive to painting, and the subcutaneous connective tissue to injections of tar, but other varieties of epithelium are less susceptible. Innumerable experiments in which tar has been introduced into various organs have yielded only an occasional carcinoma. The way in which these exceptional neoplasms are initiated remains obscure for they cannot be regularly evoked, and it can be said with no fear of contradiction that columnar epithelium and, in fact, the epithelium of glands in general, is wholly refractory to tar. In this respect the agent is strikingly analogous to X rays.

It was evident from the very first that the length of the tarring period is of decisive importance. A certain number of paintings is prerequisite to success; in the mouse, for example, at least 50 spread over 4 months. Nothing is gained by concentrating these in a shorter interval for the poisoning brought on by the large amounts of tar absorbed kills many of the animals, and in any case the tumors appear no earlier.

When the necessary total of applications has been made there is no advantage in continuing; cancer will surely arise after the lapse of the latent period. As the number of paintings is reduced the yield of tumors grows smaller and the latent period longer, another remarkable similarity between tar and radioactivity.

Microscopic examination of the lesions educed by tar has furnished information that never could have been provided by the tumors of man. This is particularly true for the initial stages of neoplasia, for in the case of the human subject one always arrives either too soon or too late. Too soon as concerns a lesion in which cancer has not yet declared itself, for there is no way of deciding whether or not it ever will become malignant; too late when the diagnosis of malignancy is certain, for then the initial stage has passed by.

With tar cancer, however, it is possible to follow every step of a process whose end is known in advance; as an instance, the significance of local circulatory changes and of inflammatory reactions in the connective tissue can be determined. Minute study of all the various proliferative stages in the epithelium has shown that tar carcinoma generally originates at several different points in the painted area. Although in theory the malignant transformation of one single cell would suffice to inaugurate cancer, in tar carcinoma at least the change involves several points simultaneously and the tumor results from coalescence of these primitive islands of neoplasia.

This meticulous study was all very well so far as it went, but differences of opinion began to arise with the attempt to go behind the scenes and discover how tar actually operates.

Casehardened adherents of the irritation hypothesis could see in it merely a common irritant, with no specific character whatsoever, that incites the malignant change only because its repeated application sets up chronic irritation. Yet nothing refutes this point of view more successfully than tar itself, for some samples are not carcinogenic at all though often more irritating than those that are so.

It appears certain, therefore, that tar has a specific carcinogenic influence, and at first it was widely believed that the effect is exerted by a direct action on epithelial cells. True, tar was known to undermine the general health of the animals for it is definitely toxic in large doses, causing degenerative changes in the liver, kidneys, spleen, and lymph nodes, but at that time no one thought them of any significance in carcinogenesis. Before long, however, it was noticed that growths may arise sometimes outside the painted area. Attacking this problem, Murphy and Sturm painted mice at a different site each time, so that no area of skin ever received enough tar to elicit a tumor though the total amount applied would have been sufficient to produce one. There were no cancers of the skin in mice thus treated, but in 60 to 78 per cent of them carcinoma of the lungs appeared. Schabad achieved a similar result by applying tar to mice in the customary way and then widely excising the painted area before cancer had emerged. In still other experiments, by Fischer-Wasels, Beck, and Oberling and Raileanu, tar was introduced subcutaneously, intravenously, or into the trachea. As a rule no tumor formed at the injection site but papillomas or cancers sometimes developed in some remote area like the skin, perhaps in burns, or in old wounds resulting from the ear tags used to identify animals by number, as in Beck's experiment and ours.

It was such observations as these that led Maisin and others to modify the early belief in the direct action of tar by suggesting that it brings about a constitutional alteration of some sort in addition to the irritative lesion set up at the point of application. The ensuing argument revolved about the old question whether cancer is a wholly local disease, like a boil, or a general disease with a local manifestation like, say, measles and its eruption. In the latter case, tar was supposed to create a constitutional change that would finally reveal itself by the appearance of a tumor, either at the place where the agent had been applied or wherever else local circumstances were propitious, as at the site of a burn, a wound, or almost any other lesion. Recent work with the carcinogenic hydrocarbons, however, has made the hypothesis wholly untenable.

Certainly there are persons more than ordinarily susceptible to a disease, tuberculosis, perhaps, or gout, who are said to have a tuberculous or a gouty *diathesis*, as the case may be, but for cancer no characteristic change in the tissues or fluids of the body has yet been demonstrated in either man or the lower animals, despite all the efforts of Reding, Slosse, and many others. Since the existence of a cancerous diathesis remains unproved, therefore, it is safer to refer the rare tumors that do appear at a site distant from the tarred region, not to any special predisposition induced by the applications, but to absorbed tar itself. Many investigators, in fact, have seen tar granules throughout the body in tarred animals, and as it is conceivable that a burn, or any other lesion, might retain these just as it might fix microbes or dyes injected into the blood stream, there need be no surprise when a tumor arises in a remote area. It is true, of course, that only minimal amounts of tar would be in play, but then such a result is by no means reproducible at will, for only an occasional animal, no doubt because local conditions are unusually favorable, reacts with the production of a distant neoplasm.

Those cancers that have developed in the lungs could easily be explained by the transport of tar from a distance to an organ in which the frequency of inflammatory bronchial lesions offers every opportunity for its fixation. But it seems, too, that in these experiments, with all their variable results, insufficient attention has been paid to heredity, an influence of the highest importance for the genesis of pulmonary cancer in mice. As recent work has shown that tar, like X rays, may reveal hereditary cancer factors, perhaps it merely augments the incidence of pulmonary carcinoma in strains of mice where this occurs spontaneously.

Research, led astray for a while, has found the highway again, but the time spent in studying remote action was not wasted. All the work seems to show that a simple inflammatory process may retain any carcinogenic agents that succeed in entering the body, and in so doing it suggests one of the mechanisms through which, in all probability, certain chronic irritative lesions end in cancer. At the moment, however, it is impossible to draw any such general conclusion, for these experiments have to do only with tar, after all, and apart from industrial cancer would apply in man only to the possible carcinogenic activity of tobacco smoke. First Roffo, then Schürch and Winterstein, and still more recently Flory, reported that tar from tobacco is carcinogenic for the rabbit and for the mouse. Now tobacco smoke, as a combustion product of tobacco, naturally contains tar, and Roffo estimated that during the lifetime of an average smoker quarts of tar may pass over the mucous membrane of his respiratory and digestive tracts. But except for this special case no one has yet been able to show that the work on tar cancer has furnished any information applicable to those neoplasms in whose production tar certainly plays no part.

It was not long, however, before investigation turned in a wholly different direction, thanks to the discovery of the carcinogenic hydrocarbons.

The Carcinogenic Hydrocarbons

In the presence of certain facts there are questions that almost ask themselves, but they are not always the easiest to answer. Tar having been proved carcinogenic, who could help wondering which of its constituents is the active agent? A difficult question, for it is composed of hundreds of chemical compounds of which most are still unrecognized, and to seek in such an incredibly complex mixture for one of these, about which nothing was known save its biological effects, was like hunting for a needle in a haystack.

Yet the task was courageously attacked. Even before the era of experimental research with tar two English investigators, Ross and Cropper, had been trying to identify the dangerous fractions with nothing to go on but chance clinical observations in man. They noticed that when coal is heated at very high temperatures, 1,000°C. or thereabouts, as in coke ovens, the resulting tars produce no tumors on the hands and arms of the workmen. Tar obtained from gasworks, on the contrary, where the coal is heated to but 800°C., is very active in eliciting warts and epitheliomas. Testing the stimulatory effect on the mitosis of white blood cells from the human subject, they came to the conclusion that cyclic hydrocarbons of the anthracene group are the mischievous element.

Now *there* was a truly remarkable feat! With observations on a relatively small number of cases and no possibility of adequately verifying their results, Ross and Cropper came very near to solving the problem.

With the introduction of a method that permitted experiments on animals the inquiry was greatly facilitated, for all the various tar fractions could be tested on mice. Foremost in this work were Bloch and Dreyfuss, Deelman, and Maisin, the result of whose various investigations was that carcinogenicity is associated with certain fractions, that the active constituent is soluble in benzol, and that it is probably a cyclic hydrocarbon of high molecular weight. They were getting closer but were still far from the goal, for the number of hydrocarbons with these properties is legion.

After these first tentative efforts, little enough encouraging to be sure, a systematic search was instituted by a man in whom patience and sagacity reached their culmination. This was Kennaway, of the Royal Cancer Hospital (Free), London, whose firm resolve it was never to give up until the problem had been solved.

The fractionation of tar is a laborious process, for every fraction again contains an enormous number of compounds. Ordinary tar is obtained by the destructive distillation of coal, and as coal itself is of highly complex and variable constitution Kennaway simplified the problem by preparing tars from substances of known chemical composition. Beginning with simple and well-known compounds like isoprene, which he heated in an atmosphere of hydrogen, he was rewarded with some highly carcinogenic tars, but even these were complex enough and testing them all for activity was a slow and troublesome job. After every new fractionation, after every attempt at further purification, the product had to be tried on mice and then came six months of waiting before the result could be known. The greatest handicap, therefore, was not material, though the number of mice used could be counted by the thousand, but time, and as the six-month periods dragged by one after another it seemed as though the solution of the problem would be postponed indefinitely.

It was then that two of Kennaway's associates, Mayneord and Hieger, had a brilliant idea. Some fractions of tar that were highly carcinogenic showed a beautiful fluorescence under ultraviolet light, and their fluorescent spectrum had three bands that seemed rather characteristic. As similar bands were found in some of Kennaway's active preparations Mayneord and Hieger suggested that this spectral quality be empirically considered a test for carcinogenicity, and that spectrographic examination be substituted for the mouse test. In other words, that instead of painting each substance on mice, an arduous task in itself, and then waiting six months for the answer, a spectral analysis be made, which, it was hoped, would provide this information immediately. Their success amply fulfilled their expectations for within a short time strongly carcinogenic compounds were obtained, in the isolation of which J. W. Cook, a chemist of the highest skill, rendered services of inestimable value. In 1930 the first chemically pure carcinogenic hydrocarbons were reported by Kennaway and Hieger, and one of the most compelling problems in all experimental medicine had been solved.

It had been realized from the first that there are many carcinogenic compounds. Only one, however, 3,4-benzpyrene, has been isolated so far from coal tar, and that by Hieger, who got 50 grams of it, not quite 2 ounces, or about the weight of 8 twenty-five cent pieces, from 2 tons of pitch. All the others have been obtained from synthetic tars, or have themselves been synthesized. The fundamental component of many is anthracene, as Ross and Cropper thought. Found in the fraction that comes over between 280° and 380°C., this is composed of three benzene nuclei.

For the benefit of those who have forgotten their chemistry it may be recalled that the formula for the benzene nucleus is C_6H_6 and that its structural formula is:

```
          H
          |
          C
        //  \
   H—C       C—H
      |       ||
   H—C       C—H
        \\  /
          C
          |
          H
```

Three such nuclei joined make anthracene:

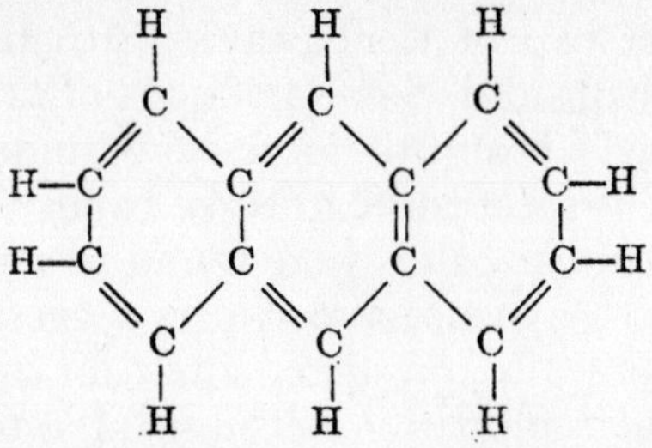

But in the interest of simplicity it is customary to give merely the hexagon and to indicate thereon only those radicals that replace hydrogen atoms. Thus anthracene would be represented as follows:

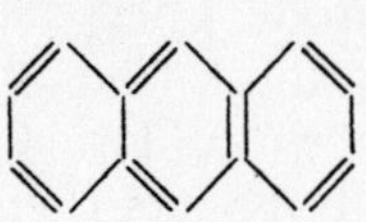

By adding another benzene ring in the 1,2 position 1,2-benzanthracene is obtained:

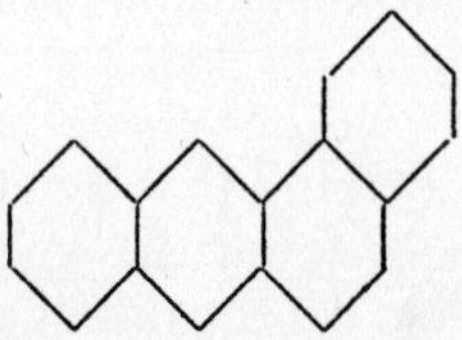

1,2-Benzanthracene is only feebly carcinogenic, but highly important for all that, because it underlies a large number of very active hydrocarbons and because in its fluorescent spectrum were found the three characteristic bands upon which Mayneord and Hieger depended for the identification of effective compounds.

The addition of another benzene ring to 1,2-benzanthracene in the 5,6 position results in 1,2,5,6-dibenzanthracene, a pentacyclic, or five-ring, compound of pronounced carcinogenic activity:

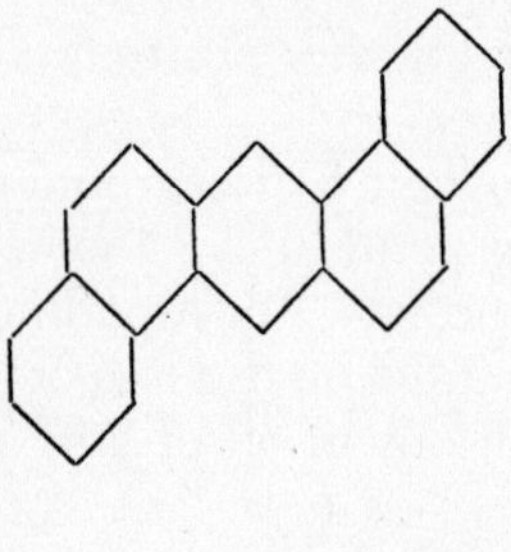

Four benzene nuclei in the following arrangement make up pyrene:

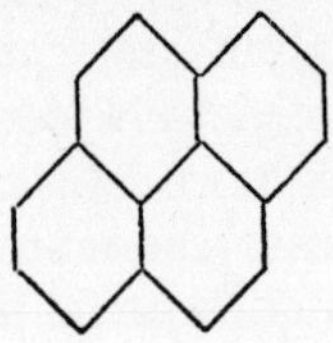

and the addition of a fifth in the 3,4 position produces 3,4-benzpyrene, one of the most active of all the carcinogenic hydrocarbons:

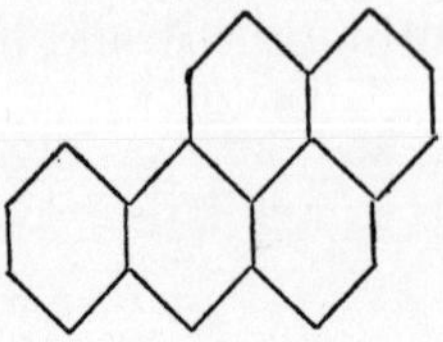

Another very important one, and a direct derivative of 1,2-benzanthracene, is methylcholanthrene:

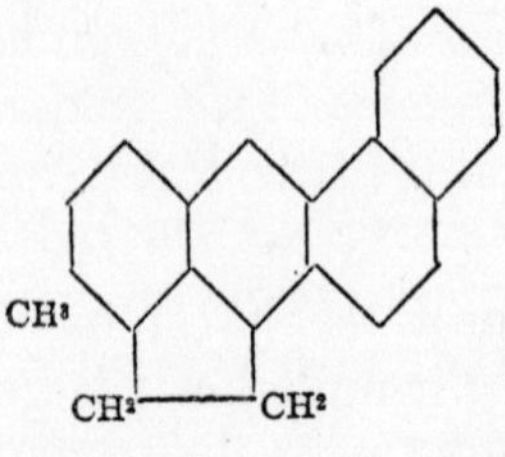

CH_3

CH_2—CH_2

The compounds mentioned are but a few of the most important among the multitude of carcinogenic hydrocarbons. The results achieved by synthesizing a large number of these substances show, here as elsewhere, the close relation between chemical structure and physiological activity, for the extensive investigations of Fieser leave no doubt that even so slight a modification as the removal of a radical or its transfer to another position is enough to withhold or confer carcinogenic power.

The synthetic carcinogenic hydrocarbons are yellowish crystals or powders with a melting point above 200°C. and soluble in benzol as well as in most oils and fats. For experimental purposes 0.1 to 10 per cent solutions are painted on the skin or injected into the various tissues and organs; solutions in oil or lard are used for administration by mouth, and colloidal preparations for introduction into the blood stream.

These are the principal results obtained. Painting elicits carcinoma of the skin in mice, rabbits, rats, and chickens, but the mouse is the animal of choice because it is especially sensitive to this mode of application. The rabbit is more resistant than it is to certain tars, an observation suggesting that there are other active agents in tar that have not yet been isolated. The rat is highly refractory to painting, and in our own experiments we had to wait two years before cancers of the skin appeared. All the tumors induced in this way have been carcinomas, usually of the squamous cell type, though in the rat we have seen basal cell carcinomas.

Injected under the skin or into the muscles the carcinogenic hydrocarbons give rise to sarcoma in the rat and the mouse, and the same variety of neoplasm has been produced in the rabbit and the chicken, but by no means so regularly.

Introduction into the peritoneal or pleural cavities, or most of the internal organs, generally results in sarcoma, though in the kidney and the prostate squamous cell carcinomas have been observed repeatedly, and Furth and Furth have caused leukemia in mice by injecting carcinogenic hydrocarbons into the spleen.

In our own experiments administration by mouth brought forth a few squamous cell carcinomas of the stomach in mice. Lorenz and Stewart obtained more interesting results, however, by giving watery emulsions of dibenzanthracene or methylcholanthrene to mice in the same way; there appeared many cancers of the lung and columnar cell carcinomas in the upper part of the small intestine. These are the first cancers of glandular epithelium to be produced by the carcinogenic hydrocarbons, but the conditions surrounding the experiment were complicated.

For one thing, the outcome was inconstant and depended largely on the strain of mice employed. For another, remote action is seen here, as in so many other experiments with these compounds, and the same question arises that was propounded in the case of tar. The effect of the carcinogenic hydrocarbons is mainly local, and where a susceptible tissue is concerned a malignant tumor invariably appears at the application site. But they can act at a distance, too, no doubt because they are absorbed and distributed throughout the body. Under such circumstances, however, the amounts involved are infinitely smaller and the results variable in proportion, for neoplasms appear only in some of the animals, depending entirely upon the strain employed, that is to say, upon hereditary factors. Beyond question the carcinogenic hydrocarbons here assume the role of revelatory condition for a cancer factor in cells that are hereditarily prepared to become malignant.

This conclusion was forced upon us in consequence of our experiments on the production of leukemia by the intravenous injection of colloidal benzpyrene into chickens. In the first series 3 out of 5 birds came down with the disease, whereas when the experiment was repeated on a larger scale leukemia arose in a single bird only out of 120. These results lead to the inference that benzpyrene excites leukemia only in fowls that are predisposed to it by certain constitutional factors. Conclusive proof of this has been furnished recently by Engelbreth-Holm and Lefèvre, who applied a carcinogen to mice of two strains bearing hereditary factors, the one for mammary carcinoma, the other for leukemia. The technic employed was that introduced by Murphy and Sturm for tar, that is, application to a different area each time to obviate the development of a local tumor. According to the strain, mammary carcinoma or leukemia, one or the other, appeared earlier and more often than in the control animals.

Similarly, both Andervont and Schabad have shown that in strains of mice predisposed to spontaneous pulmonary tumors the incidence of these growths can be increased from some 5 or 10 per cent to between 36 and 94 per cent by treatment with dibenzanthracene. Thus although the principal effect of the carcinogenic hydrocarbons is exerted upon the connective tissue and the epithelium of the skin at the application site, these compounds may influence remote tissues also, revealing hereditary factors for neoplastic processes of quite another kind, such as pulmonary and mammary carcinomas, leukemia, and so on.

In all this we can hardly fail to notice a close similarity between the carcinogenic hydrocarbons and the various forms of radiant energy, but particularly the X rays. These, too, attack by preference the surface epithelium and the connective tissue, and play the role of a revelatory condition for hereditary factors by inducing a wide variety of tumors as different mouse strains are selected for radiation.

Perhaps the analogy will be explained when we understand better how all these agents act. In the meantime, two facts seem to be well established. First, weak concentrations of the carcinogenic hydrocarbons inhibit the metabolism and mitosis of cells growing in vitro. So pronounced is this retarding effect, indeed, that certain investigators have actually tried these compounds in the treatment of

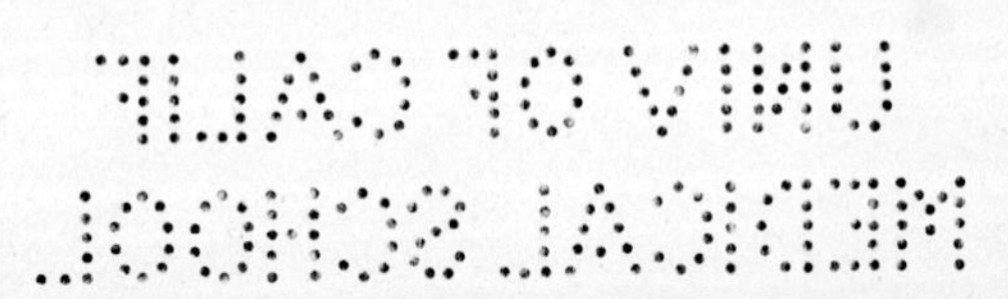

cancer, and it is equally paradoxical that the X rays, which will incite malignant growth, should be numbered among our most valuable remedies.

Secondly, the carcinogenic hydrocarbons sensitize cells to light. When the microscopic organism, paramecium, is exposed to ultraviolet radiation it suffers no evident change, nor does sojourn in a medium containing traces of a carcinogenic hydrocarbon appear to inconvenience it. But if it be exposed to ultraviolet light after having been kept for a time in such a fluid, it quickly dies. Here, as in the preceding instance, we are vouchsafed a glimpse into the relation between the electromagnetic radiations and the carcinogenic hydrocarbons.

The great value of the carcinogenic hydrocarbons to the experimentalist lies in the accuracy with which they can be administered, for when they are given subcutaneously the precise amount is known. A few milligrams (a milligram is about 1/70 of a grain) are enough to produce sarcomas regularly in the rat or the mouse within a period that varies according to the activity of the compound employed. With adequate doses it is 2 to 3 months for methylcholanthrene, 3 months for cholanthrene, 3 to 4 months for benzpyrene, and 6 to 7 months for 1,2,5,6-dibenzanthracene. With less than the optimum amount individual differences begin to appear, the number of tumors decreasing proportionately while at the same time the latent period grows longer. When the dose is considerably increased, to 75 milligrams in experiments that my associates and I carried out on the rat, the latent period is shortened but cannot be reduced below an average minimum of 2 months. The tumors develop promptly, and differ from those customarily observed not only in this rapid emergence but also in their aggressive character, which is shown by the frequency with which they metastasize.

In experiments designed to find out how small a dose would still be successful we discovered that 0.1 milligram is wholly effective, but this lower limit has been far surpassed by Shear. Using 1,2,5,6-dibenzanthracene dissolved in cholesterol he was able to elicit a subcutaneous sarcoma in a mouse with less than 0.0004 milligram. The diagnosis was confirmed by the fact that this tumor could be transplanted. Thus it is safe to say that in susceptible animals the threshold dose, the amount, in other words, that will just produce an effect, is as small as that obtaining for the hormones.

Beyond any doubt the most important outcome of all this work is the information that has been assembling on the chemical nature of the carcinogenic hydrocarbons.

Tar cancer, it must not be forgotten, was the starting point, and at first the problem was circumscribed; the desire was merely to identify the active agent in tar. But the multiplicity of effective compounds discovered, and above all the fact that only one among them had been found in tar, proved clearly that the question is much more widely inclusive. For when it was realized how many carcinogenic agents there are, nothing seemed more reasonable than to suppose that they are responsible not only for industrial cancer but for malignant neoplasms in general, and even to ask whether the body itself might not produce such compounds under abnormal conditions.

An indication that this might be so was afforded by methylcholanthrene. Most powerful of all the carcinogenic hydrocarbons so far discovered, this can be made from cholic acid and desoxycholic acid, normal constituents of the human bile. Moreover, it is chemically related to the sterols, a group of compounds highly important to the living organism that includes vitamin D, the sex hormones, and other essentials.

Entirely new prospects open before our eyes and we begin to descry some connection between the carcinogenic hydrocarbons and certain chemical compounds whose significance for the inception of malignant growth has become clearer and clearer during the past few years.

Consider first the sterols of the skin. It is known that under the influence of the ultraviolet rays one of them, ergosterol, is transformed into vitamin D, and Roffo has shown that when animals are exposed for some time to the sun another sterol, cholesterol, is notably augmented in amount. As this increase of cholesterol in the skin regularly precedes the outbreak of cancer due to ultraviolet radiation, is it not tempting to imagine that under these conditions a portion of the sterols is changed into a carcinogenic hydrocarbon? The hypothesis is still unproved and the chain of events more complex, perhaps, than we realize, but at least some connection has been established between the sterols, the carcinogenic hydrocarbons, and electromagnetic radiations that ultimately will explain the curious analogy between tar and radiant energy mentioned in preceding pages.

Again, we are beginning to detect relationships between the carcinogenic hydrocarbons and the sex hormones, especially folliculin, relationships that are mainly chemical though physiological, too, in part.

Folliculin is a generic term for the estrogens, compounds that excite estrus, or heat, thus preparing the female genital organs for impregnation and implantation of the fertilized ovum, and it has been found that some carcinogenic hydrocarbons share this property. True, they are ten to twenty thousand times less effective than folliculin, but Cook, Dodds, and Lawson have found that slight modifications in their composition confer a much higher activity.

Conversely, the estrogenic hormones may display carcinogenic power, given suitable conditions, as Lacassagne was the first to demonstrate. Leo Loeb had proved in 1919 that excision of the ovaries prevents the appearance of mammary carcinoma in mice if performed before the fourth month; after that age castration merely lowers the incidence, and beyond the seventh month has no effect at all. It is well known, too, that even in mouse strains where cancer of the mamma attacks all the females, or nearly all, the males are exempt. Thus the normal absence of folliculin in the male and its suppression by early castration in the female accomplish the same effect, and it is only reasonable to infer that this hormone plays some part in the production of mammary carcinoma.

This was conclusively proved by Lacassagne. Mice of various strains were injected weekly with estrogens from birth until they died, with different results in different strains. In those with a high rate of mammary cancer the incidence was definitely increased, the neoplasms appeared much earlier than usual, and, most interesting of all, cancer developed in the males as often as in the females. In strains that were not subject to cancer the injections did not evoke it, even in the females. On the other hand, mice treated from birth with large doses of testosterone, the male, or testicular, hormone, were definitely protected against cancer, none of the females of a highly susceptible strain having been attacked. The testosterone, acting through the pituitary gland on the ovaries, caused atrophy of their follicles; it is the antagonist, therefore, of folliculin.

The prolonged administration of estrogenic hormones to males is generally followed by atrophy of the testes, but Bonser and Robson have recently stated that in certain strains of mice the glandular portion persists, probably because the interstitial cells of Leydig, source of the male hormone, undergo considerable hyperplasia. In some cases this response may be so pronounced as to result in benign or even malignant neoplasms of these cells.

Lacassagne's findings have been confirmed by Burrows; by Gardner, Smith, Allen, and Strong; and by many others, and Geschickter has asserted that they apply equally to mammary carcinoma in the rat.

What happens here comes to pass in a manner discussed on preceding pages. Mammary cancer in the mouse depends upon a hereditary factor, but this does not become effective without the coöperation of an estrogenic hormone.

Its action in such cases can be accounted for in two different ways. Either the cells of the mammary epithelium in predisposed animals are especially sensitive to its stimulation and the hormone provokes the malignant change directly, affecting them as sunlight affects the susceptible cells in xeroderma pigmentosum; or the mammary epithelium reacts abnormally, retaining the hormone and transforming it into a carcinogenic hydrocarbon.

Whichever it may be, follicular hormone is capable of a direct carcinogenic effect, for in 5 of Lacassagne's mice sarcomas developed in the subcutaneous tissues at the injection site, an observation that has been substantiated by other investigators. Painting, however, has produced no tumors of the skin.

But the prolonged application of folliculin to the skin may elicit neoplasms in the pituitary gland, according to Cramer and Horning, and its repeated injection may cause epithelial hyperplasia in the uterus or prostate, sometimes with the subsequent appearance of lesions resembling carcinoma, as in the experiments of Pierson; Selye, Thomson, and Collip; and Overholser and Allen. Allen and Gardner, finally, in some recent experiments, have succeeded in producing cancer of the uterine cervix in 15 out of 24 mice injected with large doses of estrogenic hormone, and the role of this agent in the genesis of a common variety of carcinoma is thus becoming more and more apparent.

Such is the story of the carcinogenic hydrocarbons, one of the most valuable acquisitions of modern science, whose discovery was the outcome of zealous and unselfish research directed toward one single end, the solution of an important problem. To spend years in seeking the agent responsible for the carcinogenic activity of tar might seem to many a labor out of all proportion to any possible reward, but the biological sciences hold surprises that may outstrip the boldest imagination. Starting in a narrowly restricted field the investigator has seen his discoveries spread from tar through the bile acids, the sterols, the sex hormones, perhaps even to radiant energy.

In the similarity of their effect the carcinogenic hydrocarbons form a highly specialized group of compounds, but the past few years have shown that in their power to incite malignant growth they enjoy no monopoly. This property they share with another family of entirely different chemical composition, the aromatic amines.

In 1895 the German surgeon Rehn reported the frequent appearance of papilloma and carcinoma of the bladder among men employed in the new and flourishing aniline dye industry. Aniline is the starting point for all the brilliant dyes that play so large a part in our modern life since they are used to color not only fabrics, paper, and indeed most of the objects by which we are surrounded, but much of what we eat as well. For although most of our foods have what we are pleased to think is their natural color this is achieved not seldom with traces of aniline dyes. Thus the properties of these compounds are of interest not only to mice and rabbits but also to the consumer himself, who for once in his life, at least, becomes the experimental animal.

As for the frequent occurrence of vesical tumors in the aniline dye industry, Rehn's observations have been amply confirmed by many successors. As with other carcinogenic agents a certain length of contact is required, but this threshold once passed the neoplasm arises sooner or later, even though the baneful influence has been withdrawn in the meantime, for cancers of the bladder have appeared 5 to 35 years after the men had left the industry.

One of the first among the various components to be inculpated was betanaphthylamine, but all experiments with this compound were fruitless. It should be explained, however, that the modern technic of experimental carcinogenesis had not yet been developed, and that it was not then realized how essential is patience in all such inquiries. The investigator has to apply a substance for weeks or months, and then wait years, maybe, for his result. Only thus did Schär, in 1930, succeed in eliciting the first tumors of the bladder with betanaphthylamine. Among 16 rabbits kept in a vapor of that compound one had a papilloma and the other a cancer. The experiment was repeated by Perlmann and Staehler, who produced 7 vesical papillomas in 70 rabbits that were injected subcutaneously with betanaphthylamine; but Hueper, Wiley, and Wolfe showed that the dog lends itself more favorably to experiments of the sort. Long-repeated subcutaneous injections of a watery solution led at their hands to papilloma or carcinoma of the bladder in 9 out of 16 female dogs in 20 to 26 months, and analogous results have recently been obtained by Bonser in both male and female dogs.

Still another carcinogenic compound has been discovered in the dye scarlet R (scarlet red, or Biebrich red). About forty years ago

Bernhard Fischer (later known as Fischer-Wasels) found that its subcutaneous injection in oily solution will elicit active epithelial proliferation that closely resembles early carcinoma, though it never goes so far as to become malignant. As the dye stimulates tissue growth so effectively it became popular as a means of accelerating the healing of wounds.

Its principal component is *o*-aminoazotoluene,

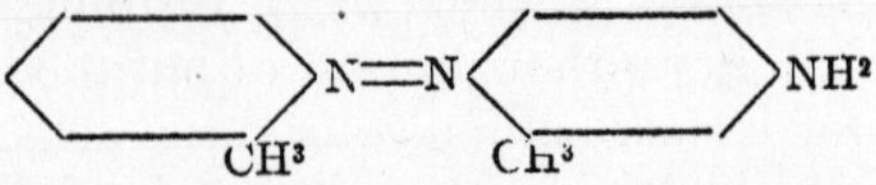

$$\text{N}{=}\text{N} \quad \text{NH}^2 \quad \text{CH}^3 \quad \text{CH}^3$$

which was isolated in 1877, but whose carcinogenic properties remained unknown until 1935, when two Japanese investigators reported their experiments. Among 360 rats fed by Sasaki and Yoshida for about a year on unpolished rice that had been soaked in an olive oil solution of this chemical, 88 died with cancer of the liver; 84 of the tumors involved the hepatic cells themselves and 4 the epithelium of the bile ducts. There was no possibility that the growths could have been spontaneous because such carcinomas are practically unknown in the rat's liver; at least, McCoy, who autopsied about 100,000 rats, and will always remain the authority on the pathology of this species, never encountered one.

The result, since confirmed in many laboratories not only on the rat but on other species as well, in the mouse, for example, by Shear, represents the first production of cancer in an internal organ by a chemical compound of known composition. But an even more active agent was soon found. This was *p*-dimethylaminoazobenzene, popularly known as butter yellow, not because it is used to color butter but because its color resembles that of butter.

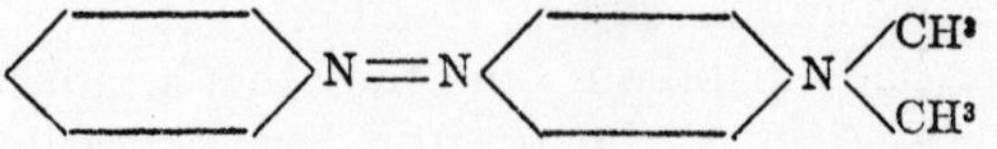

$$\text{N}{=}\text{N} \quad \text{N}\langle^{\text{CH}^3}_{\text{CH}^3}$$

In 1937 Kinosita reported that rats fed on unpolished rice soaked in a solution of this substance developed cancer of the liver in a much shorter time, and subsequently stated that there was a higher yield of these neoplasms when polished was substituted for the unpolished rice. A bread diet, on the other hand, reduced the percentage of success.

Investigators had been impressed from the very first by the dependence of these carcinomas on diet, and most of those (Okada; Ando; Nakahara, Mori, and Fujiwara; Sugiura and Rhoads; and Miller, Miner, Rusch, and Baumann) who repeated the experiment concentrated their attention on this. It was soon shown that yeast is particularly effective, since a diet containing 15 per cent of it is almost completely protective, but it may be said in a general way that partial exemption at least is conferred by any adequate diet, and that the defensive elements are above all the proteins, and vitamins of the B complex, particularly riboflavin.

The list of carcinogenic compounds is not yet complete, however. In 1936 Browning, Gulbransen, and Niven discovered in the course of a chemotherapeutic investigation that the dye styryl 430, a quinoline derivative, will elicit sarcoma in the mouse.

Not long afterward a very curious result was reported by Suntzeff, Babcock, and Leo Loeb. These investigators injected mice repeatedly with a dilute solution of hydrochloric acid adjusted to pH 5 by means of acid potassium phthalate. Of 8 mice thus treated 4 had sarcomas 10 to 16 months later at the site of the injections.

While long-continued application is under discussion it may be remarked that many surprises no doubt lie ahead of us, and that by the use of this technic we shall probably succeed in producing malignant new growths with the most unexpected substances. For instance, both Takizawa and Nonaka have elicited sarcomas in the rat and the mouse by the prolonged subcutaneous injection of strong sugar solutions, 20 to 25 per cent in strength.

Such wholly unanticipated results as these have been cited because they have a logical place in this section on the induction of malignant growths by chemical agents. But really it would be impossible to include either hydrochloric acid or sugar in the group of carcinogenic compounds that we have been discussing, and it seems highly probable that their long-continued injection must modify the tissues in some way that favors the intervention of an unrecognized carcinogenic agent already present in the body. Perhaps we should be tempted to accuse chronic irritation were it not so well known that almost indefinitely repeated injections of insulin or morphine, for instance, never of themselves result in sarcoma.

No doubt the experiments of Michalowsky are to be interpreted in the same sense. Here teratomatous tumors were evoked in the testis of the cock by injections of zinc chloride, a result that has been confirmed by Anissimova, as well as by Falin and Gromzeva, the latter of whom produced the same effect with zinc sulphate. Almost certainly the chemicals employed did no more than to produce a localized tissue necrosis, which in turn supplied the condition necessary for the participation of some other influence that alone was the culprit. Finally, in a somewhat similar experiment, Champy and

Lavedan inaugurated tumors of the testis in birds by partial castration.

The investigation of the carcinogenic compounds, at first confined to chemicals with a certain similarity of pathological action, has led gradually to other agents diverse in the extreme and wholly unlike the members of the original group, and beyond question the list will be augmented in the future in both length and variety. At the present time it appears that their action must be entirely dissimilar and that they must intervene in different phases of carcinogenesis.

In the first rank stand those that may be described as specific and unconditioned. Applied in suitable doses to a susceptible tissue these invariably lead to malignant growth with no outside aid, setting up most of, or all, the cellular changes that finally end in cancer. These same compounds, unconditioned in the case of some tissues, may be conditioned in the case of others; that is, able to bring about the malignant change only if the cells are prepared for their advent by a hereditary factor. Then, finally, there are those substances that can provoke a malignant growth only by setting up a state that is favorable to the intervention of another factor, still unknown, that is present in the body but incapable alone of acting on healthy cells. It is evident that the agents in this group may be entirely destitute of any specificity whatsoever, and probable that even injury may on occasion play the accessory role.

Rous and Kidd, in their meticulous investigation of carcinogenesis on the tarred ear of the rabbit, have contributed some interesting observations to this subject. After several months papillomas arise that will vanish if the applications are stopped. A resumption of painting elicits new crops of warts that develop more promptly than the first lot, and if these intermittent courses of tarring be continued cancer will eventually appear. But the malignant potentialities of the early changes are not manifested immediately, for if the applications be stopped in time the malignant transformation may be held in abeyance. Carcinoma will emerge, as has already been said, if painting be continued, but by then tar no longer has a specific action. It becomes merely a common irritant that may be replaced by simple traumatism.

These experiments provide a clearer insight into the role of chronic irritation. It may end in cancer when it is set up by carcinogenic agents such as tar, X rays, or hydrocarbons; or create circumstances that are favorable to the action of a carcinogenic influence; or release a carcinogenesis that has already been virtually completed.

Berenblum, who investigated the relation to carcinogenesis of the various forms of irritation elicited by diverse physical and chemical agents such as ultraviolet rays, croton oil, turpentine, xylol, and so forth, found that certain types definitely facilitate the effect of carcinogenic hydrocarbons whereas others retard it, and he attributed to this inhibition the fact that some extremely irritating tars do not give rise to malignant growths.

Such facts as these clearly prove that chronic irritation actually does play a part in the etiology of malignant growth, but at the same time they show how seriously the irritation hypothesis erred in announcing irritation as the sole cause.

Before this section is brought to a close some space should be devoted to the role played by chemical compounds in cancer of the human subject.

As man is sensitive to tar it is logical to suppose that he is equally so to the carcinogenic hydrocarbons, and the assumption is supported by recent accounts of cancer of the skin in persons who have handled them carelessly. But we should like to know also whether any malignant tumors of the internal organs are attributable to chemical agents. To answer this question a systematic search for carcinogenic compounds in the bodies of cancer patients has been started. It is known that carcinogenic hydrocarbons injected into animals are partly eliminated in the urine, where they can be detected by spectrographic methods, and with this as a basis Sobotka and Bloch examined the lipids extracted from five hundred gallons or so of urine from cancer patients, but found no trace of such a compound.

Though this inquiry led to nothing results have been achieved with an entirely different method by Schabad, who employed extracts of livers from cancer patients. This organ was chosen for several reasons. If carcinogenic hydrocarbons are manufactured in the body the best place to look for them would be the principal seat of metabolism. Then, again, the liver elaborates the bile acids, whose close relationship to methylcholanthrene, one of the most powerful among all the carcinogenic agents, has been clearly established.

With extracts prepared from the livers of cancer patients Schabad, and later Kleinenberg, Neufach, and Schabad, obtained some sarcomas at the injection site in the mouse and a definite increase in the number of neoplasms in the various organs throughout the body: mammary gland, liver, kidney, and lung. But curiously enough a few tumors were produced also with similar preparations from persons who did not have cancer. Sannié, Truhaut, and P.

Guérin have confirmed these findings, except that they saw no tumors in mice injected with liver extracts from persons without cancer.

Des Ligneris, Hieger, and Steiner have all had results entirely conforming with those of Schabad; that is to say, malignant tumors were elicited by extracts of livers whether or not these came from cancer patients. The experiments of des Ligneris are of special interest because he applied his preparation to the skin and succeeded in evoking papillomas and carcinomas in the painted area. Finally, Kleinenberg, Neufach, and Schabad showed not so long since that extracts of lung are at least as effective as those of liver.

It can no longer be doubted that the human body contains carcinogenic principles which, to judge from the method by which they can be extracted and from their biological activity, may well be related to the hydrocarbons discovered by Kennaway, Cook, and their collaborators, and chemistry will no doubt identify them in a not too distant future. The most puzzling feature about these experiments is that equally active agents are found also in persons who are free of cancer. Perhaps they might eventually have fallen victim to the disease had they lived long enough, or perhaps the absence of hereditary or other factors prevented it from developing.

The simple unvarnished truth is that we know absolutely nothing about all this, and it is humiliating to close the section in the role of an author who has written a detective story and forgotten to reveal the name of the criminal. Cancer research is face to face with a problem whose solution may direct it into channels entirely new; the issue is important, for this time we deal actually with cancer in man himself.

THE CARCINOGENIC VIRUSES

To most people microbes are the smallest possible living things. They cannot be measured in the units that we employ in our everyday life, for this would be like measuring familiar objects with a ruler about a mile long. Bacteriologists, therefore, take 1/1000 of a millimeter as a unit, which they call a *micron* and denote by the Greek letter μ (*mu*). It is equivalent to 1/25000 of an inch. The tubercle bacillus, as an example, is a slender rod 3 μ long, and some 330 of them would have to be placed end to end to equal one millimeter, or about 1/25 of an inch. In other words, if we could shrink to the size of a tubercle bacillus a millimeter would seem to us like 600 meters, or nearly half a mile.

Well, there are beings much smaller, in comparison with which microbes are veritable giants. So once more we change our yardstick, for even 1/1000 of a millimeter would be a great deal too long, and now we use the *millimu* (mμ), or *millimicron,* 1/1000 of a micron, or 1/1000000 of a millimeter.

These diminutive things are the viruses, and highly important they are for they cause serious disease in plants, the lower animals, and man.

In the human subject alone they are responsible for about thirty, among them poliomyelitis, encephalitis, rabies, smallpox, vaccinia, herpes, measles, and yellow fever. In the lower animals they cause epizootics, rapidly spreading and widely distributed disorders like cattle plague, foot-and-mouth disease, fowl plague, and many others. Some of these are so contagious and destructive that viruses have been charged, and perhaps not unfairly, with the extermination of whole species. Among plants they are an important cause of disease, and investigations of the past few decades have furnished information of the greatest interest. Here they are generally associated with destructive lesions that are characterized by a pale spotting or mottling of the leaves, whence these are called *mosaic diseases.* The microbes, even, are not spared, and by a just retribution they become victims themselves of highly contagious and fatal diseases when attacked by certain viruses called *bacteriophages.*

The viruses are intimately connected with the problem of cancer, but before we look into this question it will be necessary to review at least some of the more important facts concerning their nature and behavior. In so doing we shall enter upon one of the most fascinating chapters in all modern biology.

General Nature of the Viruses

The idea that there might be microbes of diminutive size occurred to Pasteur when he failed in all his attempts to find the organism that causes rabies, but for many years invisible microbes continued to be "creatures of the imagination," as Roux called them. Only with the experiments of Iwanowski and of Beijerinck on tobacco mosaic and those of Loeffler and Frosch on foot-and-mouth disease was their existence proved. These investigators found that the cause of the disorder, which was present in the juices of affected plants or fluid from the blisters of foot-and-mouth disease, would pass through porcelain filters with pores fine enough to hold back all microbes. The pathogenic agents must be smaller, therefore, than any known microbe, and since they reproduce themselves indefinitely, minute as they are, in an infected animal or plant, must be capable of multiplying and hence endowed with life.

Similar principles were subsequently found in a whole series of other infectious disorders, for a way of demonstrating their presence had been discovered. When an emulsion of diseased tissue is passed through a bacteriological filter any microbes or cells and cell fragments that it may hold are retained. If the clear filtrate that comes through produces the same disorder when it is inoculated into animals or plants, as the case may be, and if the process can be repeated again and again, the conclusion may be drawn that the disease is caused by an agent smaller than the microbes. Passage through appropriate filters accordingly became the principal criterion for a group of microorganisms to which the name *filterable viruses* was soon to be applied.

This standard, however, is not absolute for nature makes no leaps, as everyone knows. Microorganisms cannot be sharply divided into two groups according to whether or not they will pass through certain filters, and in reality there is a series of infinite gradations running uninterruptedly from the largest of the microbes at one end down to the smallest of the viruses at the other.

Nevertheless, one of the chief characteristics of the viruses is their small size, which makes them completely invisible even at the highest magnifications of which our very best modern microscopes are capable. In their presence, therefore, we are as though attempting to study microbes without a microscope.

Yet in various ways their shape and size have been established.

It occurred to Borrel that viruses could perhaps be made visible with a method employed by dyers in coloring fabrics. The cloth fibers are impregnated with a solution of a suitable metal and then of a dye, and the dye and metal combine to form an insoluble colored precipitate called a *lake*. A minute granule such as a virus particle, thus surrounded by a rim of lake, might be increased enough in size, thought Borrel, to be seen under the microscope, and indeed the method did expose the viruses of vaccinia, herpes, and avian molluscum as swarms of granules crowding the infected cells. It was successful with these large ones that are just on the edge of visibility, but most of the viruses are so small that they remained invisible even after the application of this special staining method.

The difficulty was surmounted by examining viruses in ultraviolet light. The magnifying power of the ordinary microscope is limited by the wave length of visible light, for if an object be smaller than half this value it will be unable to obstruct and reflect light, hence will be invisible, and since the average length of visible light waves is 550μ nothing smaller than .27μ can be seen. But the wave length of ultraviolet light is much less than that of visible light, and for this reason its use extends the limits of visibility.

It has, however, two inconveniences. It is absorbed by glass and thus will not pass through the lenses of an ordinary microscope; quartz lenses must be used. Secondly, ultraviolet light is invisible to the human eye, so there would be no point in looking through an ultraviolet microscope; nothing but black would be seen and the eye must be replaced by a photographic plate. This introduces still another difficulty, for as the image cannot be seen it must be focused in violet light, which is visible, and adjustments made for the ultraviolet. Even so it is necessary to take many photographs of an object in order to get one that is reasonably clear.

But the limit of visibility attained after all this trouble hardly goes below .12μ, inadequate for morphological investigation of the viruses since most of them are considerably smaller than this. It will be necessary, therefore, to await the perfecting of an instrument based upon an entirely different principle, the electron microscope. Instead of light rays this employs cathode rays, negative particles of electricity that stream out in a vacuum tube and have wave lengths 1,000 to 100,000 times shorter than those of light. Naturally glass or quartz lenses would be useless here, because they will not focus streams of electrons as they do light rays. The lenses of the ordinary microscope are replaced, accordingly, by coils of wire carrying an electric current that excites a magnetic field, in which the beam of electrons can be made to converge exactly as light rays are focused by lenses. For this purpose the image is received on a fluorescent screen, which makes it visible, then the screen is replaced by a plate and the image photographed. The whole apparatus has to work in a vacuum, of course, which is kept up by a mercury pump. The principle underlying it is highly ingenious and the instrument holds out immense possibilities, for magnification can be carried to an almost unlimited degree. Its use on living material has been beset by a number of difficulties, but one by one they have been vanquished and photographs of many viruses have already been obtained. These show, for example, that certain virus particles are not perfectly spherical, but somewhat elongated.

From these photographs it was a simple matter to determine the size of the particles, but it is only fair to say that the problem had been solved by then with indirect methods. Of these the most important was filtration. At first sight nothing would appear easier, given a series of filters with pores of known size, than to determine the dimensions of minute particles by employing the elementary principle of the sieve, which passes objects smaller than its meshes and holds back those that are larger. It works well enough with such things as sand, for example, but with minute particles the problem takes on an entirely different aspect, for forces now begin to intervene that may be more decisive than mere particle size.

First there is the matter of electric charge, which, already appreciable with the microbes, becomes still greater with the viruses. If the charges on the virus and the filter are opposite, one negative, the other positive, the virus will be retained even though the pores be large enough to let it pass through. Adsorption also plays a part, and both depend upon the characteristics of the fluid that contains the virus, upon its viscosity, its pH (acidity or alkalinity), and so on. Finally comes the great problem of the filters themselves. Those commonly employed by the bacteriologist and made of porcelain or kieselguhr (diatomaceous or infusorial earth) have pores of very unequal size. They may serve a rough general purpose such as ridding a fluid of microbes but they are utterly unable to furnish any precise information concerning the size of the particles that they pass or hold back.

To escape all these inconveniences and difficulties investigators had recourse to collodion membranes, the preparation and calibration of which we owe to the long and patient experiments of Elford and his associates. The method of preparation, with all the details of its exacting technic, need not be gone into here. For our present purpose it will be sufficient to know that collodion is dissolved in a mixture of alcohol and ether in the customary way, and that the size of the pores is regulated by the addition of acetone or amyl alcohol in appropriate amounts. The collodion solution is then poured out in a thin layer, allowed to solidify by evaporation of the solvent, and immersed in water. The membrane thus obtained is the filter, and with this procedure it is possible to make a graded series with pores whose diameters can be ascertained by actual measurement to run from 10 mμ up to 1μ or more.

These filters have given valuable indications respecting the size of virus particles, which are the more deserving of confidence because they have been controlled and confirmed by an entirely different procedure, namely, ultracentrifugation.

Everyone must be aware that solids suspended in a liquid can be thrown down by centrifugal force. The rapidity with which they settle depends partly upon the degree of this force, partly upon the viscosity of the liquid, but above all upon the mass of the particles in question, and this can easily be calculated when the other factors are known. The great difficulty in determining the size of virus particles by this means has been to design a centrifuge that would spin fast enough to throw down such small bodies, but the problem has been solved and apparatus is now available that will attain 30,000 to 90,000 revolutions a minute and precipitate even the finest particles.

These two procedures, ultrafiltration and ultracentrifugation, have furnished precise information on the size of virus particles, which have been found to vary within wide limits, the extremes being represented by the virus of foot-and-mouth disease with a size of 8 to 12 mμ, and that of vaccinia, which attains 200 mμ. Thus it may be said that in respect to dimensions the smallest viruses approach some of the large molecules, hemocyanin (24 mμ), pseudoglobulin (6 mμ), or hemoglobin (4 mμ). On the whole viruses must represent, therefore, agglomerations of several molecules, though there is no reason to deny the possibility that there may be virus particles consisting of but a single molecule.

Another characteristic feature of the viruses is their inability to grow on the ordinary media used for the cultivation of microbes. With a few rare exceptions these will thrive outside the body on inanimate nutritive media, upon which they can multiply indefinitely, but for the viruses no such method has yet been found. It is true that they can be preserved in active condition for several years, retaining their virulence, if the infected tissues be dried and kept in the cold, but they never multiply. This they are able to do only in a living cell, a characteristic to which the name *biotropism* has been given.

Yet they will not multiply in any cell at all without discrimination. On the whole they show a remarkable affinity for certain species of animals or plants, and within the body of a susceptible member of that species for certain kinds of cells. This attribute, known as *cytotropism,* differs in degree with each virus. That of rabies, for example, will affect a great many species, from man all the way down to the turtle. The virus of herpes attacks man, the monkey, the rabbit, and the mouse. Others, on the contrary, like that of poliomyelitis and those of certain tumors, are restricted to a single species, or nearly so. Inside a species, again, there are degrees of individual susceptibility that play an important role in the pathology of virus diseases. The investigations of Webster on St. Louis encephalitis have shown that receptivity in the mouse is associated with a constitutional hereditary factor, and a similar situation has been apparent for a long time in respect to plants. Thus certain varieties of potato are always found infected with a mosaic disease whereas others are not.

Cytotropism, indeed, is one of the most striking characteristics of the viruses. Borrel was the first to insist on this, and showed that the specificity is connected with the nature of the susceptible cells. He combined under the term *epitheliosis* such diseases as smallpox, vaccinia, herpes, and avian pox, all of which are characterized by localization of the virus in the skin. Levaditi maintained that the localization of viruses is associated with the embryological origin of the various tissues, and that there are *ectodermotropic* viruses, corresponding with those that excite the epithelioses of Borrel, *mesenchymotropic* viruses like those that cause the inguinal lymphogranuloma of Nicolas and Favre and the sarcomas and leukemias of birds, and *neurotropic* viruses, like those of rabies and poliomyelitis. In conformity with the common embryological origin of the surface epithelium and the nervous system, there are *neuroepidermal* viruses, which attack both these tissues at once.

For many viruses the cytotropism is the same, whatever the species. The virus of rabies invariably affects the nervous system, herpes virus the skin or other squamous epithelium, whence the conclusion that tissue specificity prevails over species specificity. But this is not always so, for a virus may attack different tissues in different species. The virus of yellow fever, for example, is *hepatotropic* in man and the monkey, causing in both species a degeneration of the liver that is the sign manual of the disease, whereas in the mouse it is neurotropic and sets up encephalitis; it even shows a tendency to be neurotropic in the monkey after a series of mouse passages. This proves that the viruses share with other microscopic organisms one of the fundamental properties of all living things, the power of adaptation. It would be superfluous to discuss whether in the last analysis this adaptation represents selection or the acquisition of new characteristics, for the same question might be asked of all adaptation. Nevertheless, it may well be suspected that selection plays an important part in experiments where millions or thousands of millions of individuals are manipulated.

In any case, the viruses are obligate parasites of living cells, as has already been explained; they can live and multiply nowhere else. But even though they live in cells, and at the expense of cells, they jealously preserve their own attributes, their own individuality, and do not behave as if they were mere cell products.

Of this there is ample serological proof. There are viruses called bacteriophages that infect microbes, and when one is added to a culture the microbes are disintegrated and ultimately dissolved while at the same time an enormous multiplication of bacteriophage particles takes place.

By injecting a rabbit with bacteriophage an antibacteriophage serum can be obtained, and an antimicrobe serum can be prepared by injecting another rabbit with a suspension of microbes. But the antibacteriophage serum will not act on the microbe that is parasitized by the bacteriophage, or the antimicrobe serum on the bacteriophage of this microbe. Again, the same microbe may be vulnerable to several bacteriophages, yet each of these will preserve its serological individuality.

The same thing is true of the viruses that prey on plants and animals. Tobacco and potato plants may be infected by the same virus, and this will be precipitated by an antiserum prepared against it no matter from which of the two it has been obtained, but the antiserum will have no effect upon the proteins of either tobacco or potato.

Just as a cell from the human subject preserves its characteristics even when cultivated for many generations in rabbit or sheep plasma, so do the viruses retain their own individuality without respect to the cell that serves them as a culture medium.

Viruses are not always able to enter even susceptible cells the minute they get into the body, fixed and definite preparatory conditions being often essential. Thus Calmette and Guérin found that the intravenous injection of vaccine virus into rabbits is without any apparent effect unless the skin be damaged beforehand. Evidently this virus is unable to penetrate healthy epithelial cells, but even the slight injury consequent on the plucking out of a few hairs caused vaccinia pustules to break out at the site, for during the mitosis that followed epilation the virus was able to make its way through cell walls up to that moment impenetrable.

Similar conditions certainly obtain for many other viruses and explain the breaking out of virus diseases in consequence of events that bear no apparent relation to the infection. If *herpes labialis* (cold sore) appear after an attack of fever or sunburn it is because these have set up lesions that are favorable to the localization of a virus already present in the body. A cold or an attack of grippe, both due to viruses, is frequently brought on in the same way; the chilling of the body that is so often blamed only prepares the soil by causing a congestion of the nasal or bronchial mucous membranes that makes them more receptive.

Once they have gained access to the cells viruses may announce their presence in a variety of ways. In many instances they cause degenerative changes that are rapidly succeeded by complete disintegration of nucleus and cytoplasm. These are the *cytolytic* viruses, and among them are included the viruses of poliomyelitis and fowl plague and, above all, the bacteriophages. In other cases the reactions in the cell pass through two distinct stages. First come such signs of increased activity as rapid growth of the cell body and repeated mitosis, then the picture suddenly changes and stimulation gives way to degenerative phenomena that terminate more or less rapidly in cell death. These viruses, which first stimulate and then destroy, constitute a large group that includes those responsible for most of the epithelioses, smallpox, vaccinia, and herpes.

To a third group are assigned those that incite cell division, the *cytostimulating* viruses, like those of leukemia and benign and malignant tumors throughout the various animal species.

The fourth group, finally, comprises the *latent*, or *inapparent*, viruses, which do not indicate their presence by any evident lesion. Of the highest importance to a thorough understanding of both the virus diseases and general pathology, they are widely distributed among the microbes, the plants, the lower animals, and in man himself. But how is it possible to discover a concealed infection? The question is fair enough, for as viruses can neither be seen nor cultivated it is not so easy at first to understand how their presence can be proved in the absence of all disease. A few examples will give the desired explanation.

When two strains of the same microbe are mixed it sometimes happens that all the members of both are dissolved by a bacteriophage that suddenly appears, though no sign of its presence had been given previously in either of the two. Occasionally only the organisms of one strain are affected, those of the other remaining untouched, but this is not the rule; both are more apt to suffer a common fate and disappear without leaving a trace behind. These *lysogenic* microbes, able to lyse, or dissolve, have been the subject of wide speculation, and there are not wanting those who ascribe the phenomenon to sudden production of bacteriophage by a microbe. The dogma of spontaneous generation has been resuscitated.

Actually, the matter is quite otherwise. The dissolved microbes carried a latent bacteriophage infection but, being accustomed to it, showed no sign of its presence. As soon as this "passenger" bacteriophage, this hitch hiker, came into contact with other microbes of the same species, however, its presence was revealed; it attacked the stranger, and in so doing acquired such exalted virulence as to turn on and rend its former host also.

Exactly the same phenomenon occurs with certain plant viruses. There are two varieties of potato, Duke of York and King Edward, that are always infected with a mosaic virus though they display not the slightest sign of disease, and Gratia has shown that the infection is transmitted from one generation to the next by the tubers. The virus can be made to betray its presence in three different ways.

1. Analogously to the situation obtaining with the lysogenic microbes, inoculation of juice from an infected plant into one of another variety, a President Kruger, for example, immediately reveals the disease, and by repeated passage in susceptible plants the virus can be so increased in virulence that it becomes pathogenic even for the plant whence it was derived, where it will now elicit typical mosaic lesions.

2. Inoculation of King Edward or Duke of York plants with another virus, particularly virus Y, which affects only the veins of the leaves, awakens the occult disease and both veins and parenchyma become infected, the latter by the virus that once was latent.

3. Serological reactions may be employed. Gratia has shown that the latent infection of the Duke of York potato is transmitted by the tubers, not by the true seeds, so that one can have infected or healthy plants at will merely by growing tubers or seeds. An antiserum prepared with the juices of an infected plant will precipitate the juice of that plant but will give no reaction with the juice of a healthy one, and conversely, this antiserum will be precipitated by juice from any plant at all that is infected with the virus.

It is by serological methods that the existence of a latent virus is disclosed in the lower animals also and in man. Any infected organism responds with the production of antibodies, even in the absence of all morbid manifestations. Its serum, having acquired the property of neutralizing or destroying the virus, has become *virucidal*, and the presence of these antibodies can easily be shown by experiment.

Poliomyelitis, for instance, can be transferred to monkeys. As the virus settles in the spinal cord transmission is accomplished by removing this structure from a subject dead of the disease, grinding it and suspending it in a watery medium, and inoculating this fluid. The addition to such a suspension of serum from a subject that has recovered from poliomyelitis inactivates the virus and monkeys inoculated with the mixture will not come down with the disease.

When this method had been perfected a virucidal agent was found in the blood not only of those who had recovered from poliomyelitis but of many persons who had never shown the slightest evidence of this disorder. These must have been infected at some time or other without having developed any symptoms in consequence, and investigation has proved that occult infections like this are far from rare. In the case of poliomyelitis they are common, so common, indeed, that they are the rule and illness the exception.

Latent infections may be revealed if the virus should betray its presence from time to time through recognizable disease, but there are certainly many that never give any hint of their existence and so escape all discovery.

Sometimes it happens, however, that they come to light as the outcome of pure chance.

One day Traub injected sterile bouillon into the meninges of some mice. The animals died of choriomeningitis and it was found that the disease can be transmitted by a filtrate. An inquiry immediately undertaken showed that of about 2,000 animals 40 to 50 per cent were carriers of a virus that causes choriomeningitis, and that the local disturbance created by an injection of bouillon is enough to transform the latent infection into a fatal disease. Furthermore, two caretakers of that laboratory unit had virucidal agents against this virus in their blood. They had been infected, beyond any doubt, but the fact became known only through an extraordinary coincidence.

Quite recently, again, it has been shown that human serum may contain a virus that causes more or less severe damage to the liver when injected into susceptible persons. The fact became known by the appearance of a peculiar type of infectious jaundice among people who had been treated with various vaccines for the preparation of which human serum had been used.

Still another unexpected encounter is represented by Virus III, discovered by Rivers and Tillett while they were conducting experiments on chicken pox. This virus, which seems to be indigenous to rabbits, is not harmful under ordinary conditions, but when injected into a new host it causes a local inflammatory reaction and a rapid rise of temperature. The tissues at the inoculation site are infiltrated with leucocytes, the epithelial cells involved are swollen, and both types of cell contain nuclear inclusions. Like a bacteriophage or the potato virus, this latent virus becomes pathogenic when introduced into a body to which it is not habituated.

Similar viruses have been found in the submaxillary gland of the guinea pig as well as in the kidney of the sewer rat, and such instances as all these suggest an astonishing multiplicity and extraordinary diffusion of these actual or potential agents of disaster, while at the same time they make us wonder how many more await chance discovery.

It should not be forgotten for a moment that our present knowledge is after all only a result of accidental encounters, of casual soundings in an ocean so vast that the facts already assembled seem but islets in a boundless main. We are beginning to see how important are these hidden incitants of disease, which cause infections to follow one after another, epidemics to come and go, and all without our being able to sense them. Yet it is certain that from now on research will provide an explanation for many morbid conditions of which the origin at present is shrouded in mystery.

Like Virus III, some other viruses produce in the nucleus or the cytoplasm of the cells they infect rather characteristic bodies of various sizes and shapes, that are easily stained with acid dyes. The nature of these inclusions, of which the Negri bodies of rabies and the Guarnieri bodies of smallpox and vaccinia are typical examples, remains a riddle though they have been under close scrutiny for many years. It is possible that they comprise millions of virus particles conglomerated by a cellular protein, but whatever they may be they are of interest because they sometimes disclose the presence of virus infection.

The investigations of the past few years have greatly advanced our knowledge of the chemical constitution of the viruses and the mechanism through which they act. Most of this work has been carried out on the plant viruses because they are easily handled, but above all because they are available in such large amounts; in certain plants with mosaic disease 80 per cent of the protein is virus.

Takahashi and Rawlins noticed, in 1935, that the juice expressed from plants with mosaic disease shows an optical phenomenon known as *birefringence of flow*. When the liquid is quiet it is optically inactive in polarized light, but luminous waves appear as soon as it is made to flow. The phenomenon suggests that the virus particles are rodlike in shape and tend to arrange themselves with their long axes parallel, like the fish in a school of herring. Such particles are not true crystals because the orientation of their molecules is two-dimensional, whereas that of crystals is three-dimensional; they are paracrystals, or pseudocrystals. Having discovered this property in the juices of infected plants and its absence from those of normal ones, Takahashi and Rawlins associated it with the presence of the virus.

Stanley applied to the juice of plants infected with tobacco mosaic the methods elaborated by Northrup for the purification of ferments, precipitating the proteins with 30 to 40 per cent ammonium sulphate and then dissolving them out separately in water of different degrees of acidity. Several repetitions of the process finally yielded a pure solution of virus, an opalescent liquid that deposited fine, needle-shaped crystals. These were highly virulent, and preserved their infectivity even through multiple recrystallizations.

Bawden and Pirie, working simultaneously on the same problem, showed that the spicules obtained by Stanley were not true crystals, because their molecules were arranged in two dimensions. Furthermore, these pseudocrystals still contained proteins from the plants that had furnished them. Perfecting their technic, these investigators were able to carry the purification still further and to obtain true crystals, and many plant viruses have been isolated since then in the form of beautiful rhombic dodecahedrons, since they had twelve faces, each with four equal sides and oblique angles.

Immediately arose the perfectly natural question whether these actually were virus or merely crystals of protein to which virus can adhere. The question was fully justified, for when ordinary proteins were crystallized in liquids containing viruses these clung firmly to the protein molecules and even penetrated the crystals themselves.

But Bawden and Pirie proved by a series of extremely convincing experiments that their crystals actually were the virus and nothing else. First, they were highly virulent, amounts running to a millionth of a milligram still having power to reproduce the disease. Again, similar crystals were obtained from different plants infected with the same virus and, conversely, could never be isolated from plants that were not diseased. Finally, it was impossible to demonstrate the presence of more than one substance in these crystals by any physical or physicochemical method.

In the present state of our knowledge, therefore, there is no escape from the conclusion that certain purified viruses may have a crystalline form.

Chemical analysis has proved that the plant viruses are nucleoproteins, but it is probable that others are more complex and contain lipids and carbohydrates.

One other highly interesting property of these crystals has been established. Exposure to X rays robbed them of all their virulence, though their physical and chemical properties suffered no apparent change. The virus had lost its power to multiply in susceptible cells and thus was no longer pathogenic, yet it was still able to excite the production of antibodies, an observation that may furnish fundamental information some day on the mechanism of functions now called vital. In any case, it is obvious that these sterilized viruses might be widely employed for protective vaccination and, indeed, this principle has already been realized in experiments carried out by Woglom and Warren, who were able to protect rabbits against the Shope papilloma virus with tumor extracts that had been exposed to ultraviolet irradiation.

In the light of all these facts, how is the pathogenic action of the viruses to be explained?

When one sees their astounding multiplication in an infected cell, ending with the formation of millions and perhaps thousands of millions of virus particles in every one, and when it is recollected that in some infected plants as much as 80 per cent of the proteins may be transformed in this way into virus, it seems as though viruses might cause disease solely by virtue of their presence. In reality, however, this is not so.

The gravity of a virus disease is not determined by the amount of virus present, but in large measure by its nature. Indeed, the wide variety of cellular lesions excited would of itself alone indicate a highly specialized pathogenic activity for each kind of virus, and as all this goes on inside the living cell we should confess anew our ignorance of definite facts in order that hypothesis and speculation may be given free rein.

There are certain analogies between the operations of the viruses and those of more familiar agents like the ferments, or enzymes. So striking is the similarity from certain points of view, in fact, that many investigators regard viruses and bacteriophages as a sort of enzyme, and a virus disease as a fermentative, or autocatalytic, process. The question is an important one and merits examination in some detail.

It is widely known, of course, that many chemical reactions are accelerated by the presence of substances called *catalysts*. The phenomenon is particularly striking because the catalyst never disappears during the reaction, but can be recovered at the end in its original condition; it seems to work through its mere presence. The action of most catalysts is not specific, a number of them, like acids or platinum sponge, being able to catalyze a great many different reactions. Others, however, are limited strictly to one; these are the *enzymes*, or *ferments*.

It was believed at first that certain fermentative reactions such as the production of alcohol from sugar are associated with the presence of living organisms like yeast, and *living*, or *organized*, ferments were distinguished from *nonliving, soluble,* or *unorganized,* ferments. Later it was realized that the activities even of yeast and other microorganisms are linked with enzymes that will continue to function after they have been separated from the living cell that gave them birth.

In general the enzymes are proteins of highly varied composition, glycoproteins, nucleoproteins, phosphoproteins, and so on, and their role in metabolism is enormously important, for they are the principal agents in both catabolism, or breaking down, and anabolism, or building up.

Many enzymes exist in the body in a preformed but inactive state. Thus thrombin, which assures the clotting of the blood, occurs in normal blood as prothrombin; pepsin is released by the cells that secrete it in the form of pepsinogen; trypsin as trypsinogen, and so forth. Enzymes possess the curious property, therefore, of changing an inactive form, *proenzyme, proferment,* or *zymogen,* into an active one. A trace of thrombin added to blood transforms its prothrombin to thrombin, and coagulation takes place; or trypsin, meeting trypsinogen, changes it into trypsin.

All the evidence suggests that the chemical structure of the proenzymes is very close to that of the enzymes, so it may be said that the enzymes have the power to transform closely analogous compounds into others identical with themselves. The process is strangely reminiscent of growth, for a minute amount of enzyme can multiply itself indefinitely, provided only that it has access to the corresponding proenzyme.

It is in this way that the multiplication of viruses has been explained.

If the assumption were correct every cell susceptible to a given virus should contain a preformed stage, a *provirus,* as it were, but all research directed toward the discovery of such a substance in plants has given entirely negative results. Nothing even remotely like the virus of tobacco mosaic has been found in the potato, yet that virus can easily multiply there.

Again, the viruses rigorously preserve their identity, no matter what the plant or animal in which they develop. Potato mosaic virus inoculated into a tobacco plant does not produce tobacco mosaic virus, but remains the virus of potato mosaic. Enzymes, on the contrary, do not always yield substances identical with themselves when they multiply, because they cannot make over any sort of proenzyme regardless of its source; their activities are limited by the chemical nature of the proenzyme in relation to species specificity and other factors. Thus when rabbit thrombin is added to chicken blood the result is not rabbit thrombin but chicken thrombin, and hog pepsin transforms the pepsinogen of birds into avian pepsin.

Hence identification of the viruses with the enzymes is unwarranted.

Viruses probably act in the same way as enzymes; that is, in order to multiply they fashion other proteins after their own image, but their sphere of activity is much more extensive for it is not limited even by the barrier of species. The chemical processes that the viruses must inaugurate, therefore, are infinitely more complicated, the changes imposed on the proteins more profound, than any realized by the enzymes.

The enormous complexity of all this is most eloquently expressed by the fact that the viruses, unlike the ferments, cannot operate alone but must have the living cell as an accomplice to carry their chemical reactions to perfection. It is not merely a question of raw materials, for certainly the viruses have been offered all the proteins that they could ever find in cells, yet they have not multiplied. Rather is it a question of equipment. In order to transform heat into motion a steam engine is required; mere burning of the fuel will supply nothing but heat. So with a virus, which, in order to split molecules and synthesize new proteins identical with itself, must have special apparatus that exists only in that marvelous laboratory called the cell. There all is in readiness for the application of surface forces, oxidation and reduction, and the thousand and one other processes essential to a chemistry as complicated as that of the proteins. Since these conditions cannot yet be fulfilled even by the most perfect modern technic, the culture of viruses outside the living cell has failed.

Up to a certain point this explains the varying behavior of viruses in the cells that they infect. If the constituents necessary for the growth of a virus depart widely from its own composition profound changes must be made, and only a small fraction of the disintegrated molecules will be used; the multiplication of the virus will entail considerable damage and its action will be principally cytolytic. If, on the contrary, material should be found that needs only slight modification less mischief will be done, the virus will be better tolerated, the cell will survive and, as is always the case when its internal equilibrium is upset, will react by mitosis. The virus will be cytostimulant.

Thus in the scale of life the viruses occupy a position definitely higher than that of the enzymes. Their ability to multiply at the expense of matter that is very different from them confers a certain independence, while at the same time it makes them incomparable agents of destruction.

Are they then organized beings, endowed with the properties of life, or only inanimate material produced by a sick cell?

Expressed in this form the question is unanswerable, for lack of a precise definition of life. The best that can be done is to describe the properties of living matter, properties that are but poorly defined at best and of which none is an absolute criterion.

Chiefest among them is preservation of individuality, coupled with the power of indefinite reproduction. This the viruses enjoy. The only debatable point is their inability to multiply by themselves, but here again we are beset by difficulties in definition. Is life not to be attributed to them merely because they need for their growth certain physicochemical conditions that are realized only within the cell? The day may come when these conditions can be reproduced artificially and viruses can multiply outside the living cell. Will their character then have changed? Will the dead arise? No, the definition of life must not be based on a mere method of reproduction, or even on reproduction itself. A mule cannot propagate his kind, but who would deny that he lives? A woman who has lost her ovaries is not dead!

Another characteristic of living matter is the power of adaptation. This the viruses possess to a certain degree, and it is perhaps one of the ways in which they differ most widely from inanimate chemical compounds.

Finally, the viruses share with most living things a high degree of sensitivity to heat, most of them being destroyed if kept at 50°C. for 30 minutes. Submitted to high pressures, they are inactivated between 3,000 and 6,000 atmospheres, whereas the enzymes can tolerate more than 10,000 atmospheres, according to Basset, Macheboef, and Wollman.

But there are some arguments, too, against ascribing autonomy and life to the viruses.

There is their ubiquity, in the first place. As some plants and animals perennially harbor them would it not be more logical, so runs the argument, to regard viruses as products of infected cells rather than as infectious agents foreign to the organism? The conception is manifestly false. Nothing is easier to imagine than a town where, because of bad hygienic conditions, all the houses are bug ridden. But no one would dream of saying that the houses made the bugs.

Secondly, it has been objected that the minute size of the viruses, running down almost to molecular dimensions, is incompatible with present conceptions of life. The answer to this is that our ideas of the nature of life are in no sense conclusive, and that if they prove false they will just have to be changed. We may be amazed to find processes so intricate as those of life going on in particles some of which are surely not much larger than molecules, but even the smallest virus does not differ in behavior from the largest, composed though this be of thousands of molecules; if the argument is to be based on size alone, where draw the dividing line between living and nonliving?

If we do not balk over questions of size, then, neither should life be denied to the viruses because they can be crystallized. After all, a crystal is but an assemblage of molecules arranged in a definite pattern and if proteins can be obtained in this form there is no reason why viruses should not share the property of crystallization.

Resistance to such chemical manipulations as precipitation with alcohol is no proof against the living nature of viruses. Those who advance the argument simply do not know that the spores of microbes and the seeds of some plants will tolerate not only alcohol in strong concentration but even acetone or carbon bisulphide (Gratia).

It may be concluded, then, that the viruses possess certain properties of living matter, but that on account of their infinitesimal size this inference has hardly more value than a philosophical speculation.

If we have appeared to labor the point it is only because, rightly or wrongly, the question whether viruses are animate or inanimate has always been closely linked with conjectures on their origin. And, indeed, the problem is of capital importance to a just conception of the virus diseases. Those who deny that viruses are alive regard them as cell products. The cell is supposed to prepare the agent of its own destruction, just as it elaborates autolytic ferments, so that a virus disease would be a sort of automatic and infectious suicide.

By a curious turn of fortune's wheel the doctrine of spontaneous generation, thought dead and buried long years since, has risen from its own ashes and there are heard today the very discussions that filled the scientific journals of Pasteur's era, only now they concern the viruses instead of the microbes. The outcome does not seem to be in doubt. No investigator has yet seen a virus spontaneously born of a cell, and all that we know of viruses cries out against the bare possibility of such a miracle.

Familiar now with the chief properties of these mysterious agents, we may ask what is the manner of their origin and what their rank in the world of living things.

However the activities of the viruses may be interpreted, their place is at the far borders of the animate. But as this frontier is defined by no landmarks their precise location is hypothetical and each will put them, as suits him best, at one or the other edge of the no man's land that lies between the animate and inanimate worlds.

It is natural enough to wonder if the viruses may not represent some sort of primitive or intermediate matter, in which the manifestations of life made their first appearance. Primitive forms of life are a logical postulate, certainly, yet in spite of all effort none have ever been revealed. Even though there were such, however, it would be impossible to include the viruses among them, at least those with which we are now acquainted, for how could viruses have existed without the cells that are so essential to their multiplication?

This possibility having been eliminated, two remain for consideration. One might believe with Nicolle that the viruses are simple forms of microbes, adapted for obligatory intracellular parasitism, and that this easy and irresponsible existence has led to a gradual suppression of all independence until, by progressive simplification, they have become mere aggregates of molecules with no resemblance to their ancestral type. This hypothesis has at least the virtue that it is not purely imaginative, since intermediate forms between viruses and the more highly organized microorganisms do actually exist.

According to another hypothesis, finally, viruses are cell fragments that have broken away and by a series of extraordinary coincidences have been able to invade other cells, there to survive, to multiply, and by passage from cell to cell ultimately to establish new races. Thus viruses would be particles of living matter, that have discovered a means of reproducing themselves indefinitely when the cells that gave them being have been dead for perhaps thousands of years.

While the study of viruses has already raised questions of absorbing interest the investigation has only just begun, for it is hardly eight years since one of these agents was first obtained in a pure state. The results that will accrue from methodical research are incalculable, and it is not at all impossible that they will far surpass those of bacteriology and pathology. Thus whereas the secret of life cannot now be sought elsewhere than in the cell, all hope of finding the answer there fades before the complexity of a microcosm so delicately balanced that it defies all investigation. Of the viruses this is not true. Having preserved or acquired a certain independence, they can be separated from the cell, purified, and submitted to inquiries that some day will disclose the chemical or physicochemical basis of their principal characteristics.

This knowledge will immediately prove to be of the highest import for the biological sciences. The enzymes, as we have seen, possess the curious property of being able to act on other substances of similar structure in such a way as to make these identical with themselves. In other words, they multiply by producing their likeness in the material that surrounds them. Comparing this process with the action of an electric current flowing in one wire and inducing another current in a wire near by, we may call it *multiplication by induction,* and contrast it with the more generally recognized multiplication by division. Multiplication by induction is probably one of the means employed by living matter to increase itself, molecular complexes of the cell fashioning others after their own image; this is the mechanism of assimilation, one of the principal manifestations of life.

Now for the first time this problem, vexatious since ever man began to wonder and to think, lies open to scientific analysis, thanks to those infinitesimal bits of living matter whose existence would never have been suspected did not certain of them bring formidable disease in their train.

Virus Tumors

We owe to Borrel the first suggestion that viruses may be the cause of neoplastic growth, a logical conclusion from his failure to discover the microbe of cancer. The problem had taken entire possession of his eager, inquiring mind, and tumors by the hundred and from all sources, animals and man, had been examined for a specific microbe. All in vain. Too critical to let himself be carried away with other bacteriologists by inadequate proofs, or to persevere in a line of investigation now so obviously destined to lead nowhere, he conceived the notion that he might be facing the same difficulties that had baffled Pasteur in his search for the cause of rabies. A virus seemed the only plausible solution.

Though it may be an exaggeration to say that a really new idea is always advanced too soon, this is literally true of the virus hypothesis. No other explanation has encountered so many obstacles, but it is only fair to say, also, that for many years only negative evidence could be mustered in its favor, and that it was defensible merely because no other offered a satisfactory interpretation. Facts to support it there were none; on the contrary, all those known vigorously refuted it.

While most of the findings on transplantable tumors were contradictory there was one thing at least upon which all agreed; that only by means of living cells can neoplasms be transferred from one animal to another. This observation discouraged completely all idea of a virus, for if one did exist it should be separable from the cells under suitable conditions and tumors should therefore be transmissible with filtrates.

But all such attempts failed until 1911, when Rous transferred in this way a sarcoma of the breast muscles in a Plymouth Rock hen. At about the same time two Japanese investigators, Fujinami and Inamoto, reported a filterable myxosarcoma, also of the fowl. These did not long remain isolated observations, for two years later Rous, Murphy, and Tytler described an osteosarcoma of the chicken that could be transmitted with filtrates. Curiously enough this growth, transferred in the absence of all cells, reproduced the structure of the original sarcoma, its causative agent producing, when brought into contact with connective tissue, not an ordinary spindle cell sarcoma but a growth that contained cartilage and bone. Soon afterward Rous and Lange reported a filterable angiosarcoma, again of the fowl, and since then many other avian tumors of various types, spindle cell sarcomas, myxosarcomas, endotheliomas, and so on, have been transmitted in the same way.

Rous's first papers aroused little interest, and as the infection hypothesis had always been vigorously opposed the general attitude was one of skepticism. The objections raised fell into two general patterns.

First, it was suggested that the lesions produced by these filtrates were unusually vigorous inflammatory overgrowths rather than real sarcomas.

Secondly, if they actually were sarcomas then the filtration could not have removed every single cell and cell fragment, for in spite of all precautions, so it was said, a few cells may pass a filter. In such a case the tumors produced by the filtrates would be but ordinary transplanted new growths after all.

Neither of these objections has been sustained.

Careful morphological examination of the various filterable neoplasms of the fowl leaves no doubt of their malignant nature, and as for filtration, constant improvements in technic have eliminated all sources of error there. Filtrates obtained under the most rigorous precautions have proved themselves highly active, and ultrafiltration has established the corpuscular nature of the agents and set the size of their particles at 100 mμ (Ledingham and Gye; Amies); thus they resemble the viruses of moderate size.

But entirely apart from this whole question of filtration, the unique nature of these sarcomas is indicated by their transmissibility after they have been dried or stored in glycerol, measures that are certainly fatal to cells. This fact, emphasized by Rous, has been verified over and over again, for pieces of tumor have been sent in this condition to various laboratories, sometimes even across oceans, with no loss in activity.

The occurrence in fowls of tumors that can be transmitted by means of cell-free filtrates can thus no longer be disputed, and their discovery marked an important stage in the history of experimental cancer research.

It goes without saying that all such growths can be transplanted by grafting; in this case evolution of the neoplasm is much more rapid because the graft immediately begins to proliferate. When a filtrate is injected the sarcoma develops slowly and the outcome is not so constant, but it may be improved by the simultaneous introduction of an irritating foreign body like diatomaceous earth. The ensuing inflammatory reaction leads to the appearance of young connective tissue cells that are eagerly attacked by the virus. Once started, the tumor grows quickly, attaining the size of a man's fist in three or four weeks, and soon causes death from cachexia or the presence of metastases in the internal organs.

At autopsy a definitely invasive neoplasm is found that is sometimes firm in consistency, sometimes soft and permeated by a gelatinous, ropy fluid. Areas of necrosis and hemorrhage are often encountered, and metastases are regularly seen in the lungs and liver in the form of well circumscribed, grayish-white nodules of variable shape and size. In addition to these white metastases the liver sometimes contains small, deep-red foci to which Pentimalli has given the name *red metastases.*

Microscopic examination discloses a sarcoma composed of spindle-shaped connective tissue cells resembling fibroblasts, and roundish elements of the macrophage type, the proportion of the two varying in different tumors and even in different parts of the same tumor.

Metastasis takes place by the emigration of tumor cells but in addition to this method of dissemination, common to all malignant neoplasms, areas of endothelial proliferation are found in the liver, corresponding to the red metastases and due beyond question to localization of the agent.

Like all malignant tumors these sarcomas in general are species specific, though heterotransplantation into closely related species such as the guinea fowl or the pheasant sometimes succeeds; the Fujinami sarcoma alone can be transmitted with fair ease to the duck.

The agent of a filterable sarcoma is definitely cytotropic, resembling in this respect the viruses. It selects unerringly the connective tissue, but even here it is young dividing fibroblasts and the macrophages that are most likely to be invaded and that permit multiplication of the agent. Although Carrel concluded from his experiments on sarcoma grown in vitro that only the macrophages carry the agent, the more recent investigations of Doljanski and Tenenbaum prove that both types of cell harbor it and assure its growth.

Its cytotropism is further evident from the outcome of intravenous injection. A tumor generally arises at the inoculation site, where the connective tissue has been damaged by the needle, but the formation of tumors at a distance is very rare, since the agent finds no opportunity to invade susceptible cells. It can localize, however, and elicit sarcomas at any site where wounds or burns are inflicted, as Pentimalli has shown.

The agent, like most of the viruses, is destroyed by heating for 30 minutes to 56°C., or by antiseptics such as formalin, bichloride of mercury, or tincture of iodine, even in weak solution. On the other hand, it is fairly resistant to X rays and by suitable doses all the tumor cells can be killed though the agent that they enclose remains unharmed, as the experiments of Peacock so clearly demonstrate. A sarcoma was grafted into one wing of a chicken and when it had reached an appropriate size was irradiated. The tumor disappeared but the agent remained and was taken up by the lymphatics, along the course of which rows of neoplastic nodules later appeared.

The etiological agent, as it is found in tumor filtrates, thus shows many analogies with the viruses. Yet it possesses some properties that distinguish it from these and that have continued to excite the interest of investigators for many years.

For example, filtrates are not uniformly active, and tolerate high dilution badly. The explanation for this has been furnished by Claude, who showed that the agent is adsorbed on the proteins of these extracts and exposed to the influence of an inhibitory substance that is always present in large quantities in the serum of sarcoma-bearing fowls.

Isolation of the agent by chemical or physicochemical measures, attempted for many years in vain, was finally accomplished by the same investigator, who employed centrifugation. By this means a highly purified fraction was achieved that produced uniform results and remained active in amounts as small as one ten-millionth of a milligram. Chemical analysis showed a complex mixture of nucleic acids, a phospholipid that is probably lecithin, and sugars.

Injection of the agent into a foreign species, the rabbit for example, excites the production of antibodies that neutralize the sarcomatogenic properties of filtrates, and with such an antiserum chickens can be immunized against the virus. But those protected in this way against filtrates are nevertheless receptive to tumor grafts. The virus, secure in the cells of the sarcoma, is beyond the reach of the antiserum, and this is the reason, too, why the injection of an immunizing serum is without any effect upon a tumor that is already established.

Like other viruses, those of the filterable sarcomas preserve their individuality even though they develop in the body of a strange species. The work of Gye and his collaborators has shown that sojourn of the Fujinami fowl sarcoma in the duck does not alter the serological behavior of its agent. The antiserum produced by a chicken-grown tumor will neutralize the virus of a duck-grown tumor, and vice versa.

Investigations of this sort have established a complete parallelism between the sarcomatogenic agents and the more wholly authentic viruses, but in spite of all this evidence of similarity there is still a widespread desire to establish differences between them at any price. Such is the opposition arrayed against the infection hypothesis.

Some have proposed that the sarcomatogenic agents are *organizers*, analogous to those discovered by Spemann in the embryo. He showed that certain embryonal tissues determine the differentiation of others that come into contact with them, certain parts of the mesoblast, for example, acting on the ectoderm to cause its invagination and transformation into the neural tube. If a fragment of mesoblast be transplanted under the skin of another embryo the ectoderm that meets it will develop a neural tube, although under normal conditions it would form skin. In this way various cell differentiations can be elicited at will and supernumerary organs created, merely by the selection and implantation of appropriate grafts. This influence is by no means confined to living cells, for a neural tube will be formed even if the fragment of mesoblast employed has been killed. Hence the organizers must be of rather simple chemical nature.

Is it possible to regard the etiological agents of the filterable sarcomas as organizers, endowed with the power to change normal connective tissue cells into malignant cells?

Several objections immediately arise. In the first place, organizers are provided by embryonal cells and act only on embryonal tissues, while the sarcomatogenic agents affect the cells of an adult organism. Secondly, organizers determine the *differentiation* of cells with which they come into contact whereas the sarcoma agents cause *dedifferentiation*; thus, as Rous has said, they are disorganizers rather than organizers. In the third place, organizers do not multiply in the cells that are susceptible to their influence. And finally, organizers are not destroyed by boiling (Holtfreter) and a large variety of chemical compounds can assume the same role; the sarcomatogenic agents, on the contrary, cannot endure a temperature of 56°C. for more than a short time and show a remarkable specificity.

The suggestion that the etiological agents of the filterable sarcomas are organizers does not withstand critical examination.

Again, Claude and Murphy have sought to identify them with a factor responsible for the transmutation of pneumococci described by Griffith; Neufeld and Levinthal; Dawson and Sia; and especially by Alloway. The proposal merits a somewhat detailed discussion.

Thirty-two types of pneumococcus are recognized at present, that differ among themselves in chemical characteristics and in virulence. The individuality of these types is associated with polysaccharides, which are elaborated by the microbes themselves and surround each as a capsule. If cultivated on certain media the pneumococci can no longer produce these sugars, and at the same time lose their pathogenicity as they do the features characteristic for their various types.

When filtered extracts of another type are added to pneumococci thus deprived of their capsules these microbes resume the production of capsules and, curiously enough, the polysaccharides of which these envelopes are composed are now identical with those of the type that furnished the extract. For example, if to type 2 pneumococci that have lost their capsules there be added an extract of type 3 pneumococci the former will produce polysaccharides characteristic of type 3. In other words, type 2 have been transformed into type 3 pneumococci, and this change is hereditarily transmitted to their descendants.

Extracts of pneumococci must contain, therefore, a substance with the mysterious power of causing the mutation of one type to another. To it Murphy has given the name *transmissible mutagen*, and has suggested that the etiological agents of the filterable sarcomas may be of the same nature.

The conception, however, immediately encounters a series of obstacles. In the first place, there is no evidence at present for the assumption that phenomena observed among beings so low in the life scale as the pneumococci may be applied to cells that are infinitely more complex in their organization. Secondly, it must be confessed that our knowledge of these mutations among the pneumococci is no more than fragmentary; practically nothing is known of the responsible substance, in fact, save that it is sensitive to heat, an observation that seems to indicate the presence of proteins in its constitution.

While the agents of the infectious sarcomas share the principal characteristics of the viruses, no such similarity has yet been demonstrated between these and the mutagen; if an analogy should some day come to light there will be great difficulty in distinguishing between viruses and mutagens. In such a case a virulent pneumococcus would be assigned the role of a microbe, harmless in itself, in symbiotic association with a virus.

But this is a scientific daydream, for which the mutagen hypothesis itself is responsible, and that is the main objection to it. A hypothesis for the future? Perhaps. But today it rests upon a foundation so insecure that it should not be allowed to supplant the infinitely safer virus hypothesis.

It has been suggested, finally, that the sarcomatogenic agents may be enzymes, elaborated by the tumor cells themselves. This is, in effect, the hypothesis that has been proposed for viruses in general and all the arguments marshaled against it in preceding pages apply equally here, yet it has been a prominent feature in discussions of the filterable sarcomas because some investigators believe they have supported it with experimental proof that cannot be gainsaid.

Their experiments were based on the following train of thought.

To decide whether a filterable agent is an exogenous virus, or an enzyme produced by the tumor cells themselves, it would be necessary only to ascertain whether sarcomas inaugurated by chemical agents are filterable or not. For if these neoplasms, in whose genesis no virus has taken part, can be transmitted with a filtrate the filterable agent must have been elaborated by the tumor cells. The first experiment of this sort was made by Carrel, and the result caused a sensation.

He deposited in the pectoral muscles of chickens an embryo emulsion that had been treated with very dilute arsenous acid (1:125,000 to 1:150,000) or indol (1:1,250 to 1:5,000). Sarcomas developed rapidly at the injection site that killed the birds after 17 to 35 days, and they could be transmitted by a filtrate; thus, although produced by chemical compounds, they behaved in the same way as spontaneous sarcomas of the fowl. Carrel therefore concluded that the etiological agents of filterable sarcomas are not exogenous viruses but substances formed within the cells of the tumor, no matter what its cause.

It should be pointed out, however, that despite numerous attempts in many different laboratories these experiments have never been confirmed. A few investigators, it is true, have obtained neoplasms by injecting fowls with hashed embryos and arsenous acid, and those described by White could even be transmitted with filtrates. But success has been rare indeed in proportion to the failures reported from almost every laboratory in which Carrel's work has been repeated. Like all experiments that use embryonal tissues in an attempt to produce malignant tumors, this one is extremely uncertain in its outcome, and there is little difficulty in believing that when a positive result is achieved it follows the intrusion of some factor unsuspected by the investigator.

As this, naturally, might be a virus, it would not be surprising if some of the so-called chemical sarcomas turned out to be transmissible with filtrates. Experiments of this nature, therefore, cannot be relied upon to furnish any information whatsoever concerning the nature of the filterable agents.

Then there may be cited the experiments of McIntosh, who elicited sarcomas by injecting tar into the pectoral muscles of fowls. Six of the tumors were transplantable and three of these, after they had been propagated for a time, proved to be transmissible with filtrates.

His experiments have been criticized, however, by Peacock, who himself had devoted several years of painstaking work to the question and out of his wide experience suggested certain sources of error that might have vitiated the result. By injecting tar into the pectoral muscles of fowls Peacock, also, had obtained a number of sarcomas, but none of them could be transmitted with a filtrate. Furthermore, these tumors, despite their structural identity with the filterable sarcomas, differed from them in several biological characteristics; they withstood neither drying nor glycerol, and did not recur after irradiation treatment as the filterable neoplasms so often do.

As these observations have been confirmed by Sturm and Murphy, Murphy and Landsteiner, Mellanby, and Rothbard and Herman, it is safe to say that the filterability of artificially induced sarcomas remains to be proved.

Still, this is a matter of no great importance. Even assuming that McIntosh's results were incontestable and that after several passages tar sarcomas actually were transmitted with filtrates, would this exclude the intervention of an exogenous virus? Should we be justified in concluding that the filterable agent is a product of the sarcoma cells themselves?

Not by any means.

The reasoning behind these experiments contains two premises that seemed twenty years ago to be supported by unassailable evidence but that are no longer valid today.

First, it is assumed that the fowls injected with tar were free of all sarcomatogenic virus, but where is the proof of this? From all that is known today of latent viruses an occult infection is readily conceivable, for as viruses are so widely distributed most chickens may very well be carriers of one that induces malignant growths.

Second, it is assumed that the tar elicited the sarcomas, but this has not been proved either. It might equally well be supposed to have produced lesions that made the cells receptive to a latent virus, which, in reality, was the cause of the sarcomas.

In any case this seems to be the logical explanation for an experiment recently described by des Ligneris, who brought about the malignant change in vitro by the addition of dibenzanthracene to a culture of chicken fibroblasts. The rapidity with which the neoplastic transformation took place suggests in itself the intervention of a virus, and the behavior of the tumors produced by transplanting these cultures, eventually transmitted with filtrates, resembled in many ways that of the Fujinami sarcoma. Evidently the cultures either were contaminated from the first with a sarcomatogenic virus, or later became so.

The filterability of a sarcoma obtained by injecting tar or a carcinogenic hydrocarbon has nothing in it of mystery, therefore, and cannot be used as evidence against the presence of an exogenous virus. This is no mere opinion, for facts are multiplying daily to render such a line of reasoning more and more plausible, and, in fact, latent infection by a sarcoma virus has been proved by the recent experiments of Duran-Reynals.

The serological investigations of Foulds and Dmochowski on chickens bearing sarcomas produced with chemical agents have given surprising results in this connection. The blood of these birds contained antibodies that neutralized the agent of filterable sarcomas, reacting accordingly from a serological point of view as does the blood of fowls with virus tumors, though these sarcomas could not be transmitted by filtrates. Andrewes, again, in a highly significant experiment, succeeded in transmitting tar tumors of chickens to pheasants. In the serum of all the inoculated birds virucidal antibodies for the causative agent of the Rous sarcoma made their appearance, though these were never found in the blood of normal pheasants. Such facts as these suggest that a tumor may be due to a virus and yet not filterable, which is, after all, exactly what experience indicates.

It must be recalled that not all filterable sarcomas can be transmitted with a filtrate at first, but only after transfer for a number of generations with grafts; thus, for example, Fujinami transplanted his sarcoma for two years before he was able to transmit it with a filtrate. Even growths whose filterability has been clearly established sometimes cannot be transmitted in this way.

The reasons are not entirely clear, but it is known that one of them is the presence of virucidal agents in the host. It has already been explained on a preceding page how a subject with poliomyelitis carries neutralizing antibodies in his blood, and sarcoma-bearing birds do the same. In neither case, however, can the antibodies destroy virus that is safely ensconced in cells, so that when these diseases have fully established themselves they pursue their course unchanged.

The existence of antibodies in the blood may come to light, however, if isolation of a virus be attempted. For instance, when a tumor is extracted for filtration its cells are first ground to a paste and, as a neoplasm always contains blood, liberated virus meets any virucidal agent that may be present. If it be abundant the virus will be completely neutralized and transmission by filtrate will fail. Inactivation takes place the more readily because the methods of filtration ordinarily employed are of necessity so slow that ample time is given for the antibodies to exert their full effect.

That something of the sort actually happens has been shown by Claude in the case of a chicken sarcoma that had been transplanted by grafting for ten years but could never be transmitted with a filtrate. Nevertheless its infectious origin seemed probable because chickens bearing it developed antibodies in their blood that would neutralize certain sarcoma viruses. Now virus particles in an extract can be separated from antibodies, and their activity thus preserved, by ultracentrifugation, for the former, being heavier, are thrown down to the bottom of the tube beyond the reach of the antibodies, which remain in the upper layers of the liquid. Application of this method to the tumor in question removed an active virus, and transmission with this fraction of the filtrate was accomplished.

In the near future other neoplasms that have stubbornly resisted all efforts at filtration will no doubt yield to some such means. The domain of the avian tumors is being considerably widened and the situation has undergone a complete change, the preponderant role of viruses becoming more evident with each passing day. Even though the transmission of chemically induced neoplasms should eventually be accomplished, by a technic that is beyond criticism, this will be no argument against the existence of sarcomatogenic viruses. On the contrary, it will indicate strongly their intervention, whereas some twenty years ago the same results would have been considered as a definite proof against the intervention of an exogenous agent.

A short account of the *transmissible leukemias* brings to a close this section on the filterable sarcomas of birds.

The leukemias are characterized by an excessive and disorganized proliferation of the cells that normally give rise to the white blood corpuscles. These immature elements, situated in the lymph nodes, the bone marrow, and the spleen, begin to multiply vigorously and produce constantly increasing numbers of young cells that gain the blood stream and little by little supplant the normal, mature corpuscles.

The duration of the disease in man is highly variable. Some types evolve with extreme rapidity, causing death after a few weeks, but the chronic form, which lasts for several years, is much more common.

As to its nature, leukemia still remains a mystery. Some authorities, impressed above all by the acute form, regard it as an infection and thus include it with the inflammatory processes. Others, emphasizing the proliferative nature of the lesions, place it among the neoplastic disorders, believing with Bard and others that leukemia is a malignant tumor of the blood.

Leukemia occurs also in the fowl, where it involves particularly the erythroblast, immature form of the red-blood cell, but apart from this peculiarity it behaves just as it does in mammals. The affected cells increase in number, permeate the bone marrow, invade the circulating blood, and gradually suppress the normal cells.

In 1918 the Danish pathologist Ellermann proved that fowl leukemia can be transmitted from one chicken to another by the injection of blood and of organ extracts, even after they have been filtered. Both show an extraordinary virulence, one one-millionth of a cubic centimeter of blood being enough to infect. The reaction of the etiological agent to various physical and chemical influences being identical with that of the sarcomatogenic viruses, the conclusion may safely be drawn that it, too, is a virus.

It shares with other viruses a preference for one certain type of cell. Injected into a vein, it disappears rapidly from the circulation and settles down in the bone marrow, where it seizes upon the erythroblasts. Its presence is soon announced by a vigorous proliferation of these elements, of which pathological forms begin to appear in the circulating blood after 8 to 15 days, and at last the blood is literally inundated with them.

Here, then, is an agent that pounces unerringly upon one variety of cell and causes its excessive proliferation. As it appeared an interesting experiment to try to direct the tropism of this virus toward cells of another kind in the hope of obtaining a malignant tumor, Oberling and Guérin made the attempt, but at first with no success. The injection of embryo emulsion before or simultaneously with the virus, the production of inflammatory foci, increasing the virulence of the agent by repeated passage through young birds, inoculating it into tissues growing in vitro, all these and many other artifices ended in complete failure. Finally, a virus was tried that had been attenuated by prolonged storage in glycerol in the icebox and this, when injected into the pectoral muscles, elicited sarcomas at the inoculation site.

The structure of these tumors was variable in the extreme. Some closely resembled the usual virus sarcoma, others were characterized by an abundant production of collagen. Certain of them gave rise to tumorous nodules at a distance from the primary growth, some of which were thought to be true metastases because of their morphological resemblance to it. Still others were of an entirely different structure: papillary outgrowths of the pericardium and the vascular endothelium, tumors of the intestinal musculature, reticulum cell neoplasms of the bone marrow, and so on. The only possible explanation for all this prodigality is a direct infection of different types of cell.

When these tumors were grafted into other chickens, leukemia reappeared. The virus evidently recovered its selectivity for erythroblasts, and the hosts were carried off by leukemia before tumors had an opportunity to develop. But when their blood was stored for a time, as before, it elicited neoplasms again, and the cycle leukemia—sarcoma, sarcoma—leukemia, could be reproduced with ease.

While these experiments, since confirmed by Engelbreth-Holm, Furth, Jármai, Storti and Zaietta, and others, illustrate the close relationship between the leukemias and the malignant growths, they really have a much wider applicability in that they disclose for the first time a highly important feature of the viruses. This is their aptitude for mutation, since the behavior of our leukemic virus can be explained in no other way. At a certain time, and under the influence of factors that remain undetermined in spite of all our efforts, the virus changes its affinity and attacks various types of cells, eliciting tumors and tissue proliferations in the greatest possible variety.

A propensity for mutation has recently come to light again in the experiments of Duran-Reynals. The Rous chicken sarcoma cannot be transmitted to adult ducks, but by injecting extracts of this tumor into newly hatched ducklings Duran-Reynals obtained neoplastic lesions of two kinds, *immediate* and *late*. The immediate tumors developed within one month after inoculation, the late ones not for several months, when the birds had reached adult age. The immediate tumors could be transmitted without difficulty back to chickens, but not to ducks; the virus responsible for them had remained a chicken virus. The late variety, on the other hand, were no longer transmissible to chickens, though their transfer to ducks presented no difficulty; during its sojourn in the duck the virus had become a duck virus. The most interesting observation of all, however, is that this mutation was accompanied by fundamental modifications in cytotropism that were reflected in the wide assortment of neoplasms induced: fibrosarcomas, osteosarcomas, giant cell sarcomas, angiomatous tumors, lymphosarcomas, and leukemias.

Before passing on to the virus tumors of mammals we should mention an adenocarcinoma of the kidney in the frog (*Rana pipiens*), discovered and described by Lucké and Schlumberger, which, as the frequent presence of intranuclear inclusion bodies suggests, may be caused by a virus. When tumor grafts were introduced under the skin or into the abdominal cavity no tumors arose at the inoculation site, but growths were often found in the kidney. As similar results were obtained with grafts that had been killed with cold or prolonged storage in glycerol, it is difficult indeed to escape the impression of a virus with selective affinity for the renal epithelium.

So, therefore, the occurrence of virus tumors in batrachians, and above all in birds, cannot be denied. As for the mammals, the innumerable attempts to transmit their neoplasms with filtrates failed so miserably as to lead in the end to the dogma that malignant tumors can be transferred only with living cells.

Here we approach one of the most controversial points in the whole vexed question of tumor viruses, one that long served as a springboard for all attacks on the infection hypothesis. Sarcomas caused by a virus, leukemias caused by a virus—that's all very well, it was said, but these have been found only in birds; when the experiment is carried over to mammals it turns out that neither disease can be transmitted with filtrates. Some went so far, indeed, as to propose that filterability is associated, not with the presence of a virus but with some special property of avian cells. Of course no one ever troubled himself to define this miraculous property, which could explain the transmission of a disease with filtrates without recourse to the virus hypothesis. The main thing was to discredit the viruses, even where their participation seemed most evident, in order the more easily to prevent the infection hypothesis from encroaching on the mammalian tumors.

For many years only argument by analogy could have justified such an invasion in any case, but facts are stronger than hypotheses and at last the boundary between birds and mammals has been safely crossed.

In 1898 Sanarelli described a curious disease that had made its appearance in a rabbit colony. It began with conjunctivitis, to which was soon added an edematous inflammation of the eyelids. Small tumors then began to arise at various points in the subcutaneous tissue, especially on the extremities and at the base of the ears, while in the meantime the edema spread to the snout, giving the head of the animal a leonine aspect. A similar edematous infiltration involved the anal and genitourinary orifices, where it produced enormous swellings, and the animals died after 2 to 5 days, terribly disfigured and repulsive to see.

The disease proved highly contagious. A trace of secretion from the conjunctiva instilled into the eye of a healthy rabbit brought on inevitably a fatal infection, and the disorder could be transferred with equal facility by inoculating blood or a fragment of an organ or of one of the subcutaneous tumors.

The absence of all microbes and transmission by filtrates soon established the etiological agent as a virus, a conclusion that was fully confirmed by later investigations, but interpretation of the lesions remained a matter of discussion for years. Microscopic examination, of the tumorous subcutaneous infiltrations in particular, revealed actively proliferating, star-shaped, connective tissue cells embedded in a mucoid material. The picture was not without similarity to certain myxomatous tumors of the human subject, and for this reason Sanarelli called the disease *infectious myxoma of the rabbit*. The name has never been taken in its strict sense, however, for the analogy rested only upon a more or less distant morphological resemblance, and the infectious origin and rapid evolution of the malady were thought sufficient to preclude any serious comparison with the true neoplasms.

In 1932 Shope described small fibromatous tumors situated under the skin of the forepaws and hindpaws in a wild, cottontail rabbit. These growths, which had the microscopic structure of a hard fibroma, could be transferred not only by grafts but by filtrates, and equally well to both cottontail and domestic rabbits. In the latter the neoplasms grew more rapidly at first, though after they had reached a certain size they began to regress and ultimately disappeared. These rabbits, in which infectious fibromas had receded, proved resistant to the infectious myxoma, but the converse test could not be carried out because the myxoma is always fatal to the domestic rabbit.

Though the wild rabbit, on the contrary, has always been considered resistant to myxoma, Shope was able to elicit characteristic lesions by inoculating it into the testis. A mucoid tissue appeared in the organ, but the disease remained localized and sooner or later underwent spontaneous cure. Then, and then only, was the wild rabbit really immune to myxoma, and it proved to be immune also to the infectious fibroma. Thus a cross immunity can be established between the two diseases, the fibroma immunizing against the myxoma, and the myxoma against the fibroma. They are a result, therefore, of related causes; myxoma is a highly virulent form of fibroma, and the analogy between the two is a little like that between smallpox and vaccinia.

A number of highly interesting facts relating to the virus tumors of mammals have been accumulated through the study of a papilloma, also introduced by Shope and obtained in wild rabbits from Iowa and Kansas.

These animals often develop new growths in more or less considerable number, generally on the skin covering the abdomen or the neck and shoulders. These appear as large warts; dry; dark; with an irregular, fissured surface; usually constricted at the base; and vertically striped, because each individual wart is composed of closely packed and almost homogeneous upright strands of tissue. Under the microscope they resemble any extensively keratinized wart.

Some of these papillomas that had been stored in glycerol Shope ground to a paste in physiological saline solution. The extract was centrifuged, filtered, and then applied to the skin of rabbits after light scarification with a needle or sandpaper. At the end of a 6 to 12 day latent period papillomas began to appear, and about 6 weeks after inoculation reached their full development. In brief, this papilloma of the wild rabbit was transmissible with filtrates, and its etiological agent answered all the tests for a virus.

Inoculation into rats, mice, guinea pigs, cats, hogs, and goats was regularly unsuccessful; the rabbit alone was susceptible. But the epithelial cells of its mouth and respiratory and genitourinary passages, despite their close resemblance to those of the skin, were completely refractory to the virus.

The tumor could be transmitted with filtrates to both wild and domestic rabbits, though it pursued a different course in each. In the former it grew slowly and ended as extensively keratinized papillomas that tended to become detached and finally regressed and disappeared. In the domestic rabbit the warts developed much more rapidly, probably because the soil is more favorable to the cytostimulating action of the virus. They were more fleshy and less extensively keratinized than in the wild rabbit, but the proliferating epithelium never invaded the underlying tissues; in their earliest phases, at least, the growths remained true papillomas.

Rous tried to direct the growing epithelium downward by covering the warts with collodion, by traumatizing or infecting the connective tissue beneath them, or by injecting irritating substances, but much more satisfactory results were achieved by inoculating tumor fragments into the muscles or the internal organs. There the cells assumed a frankly invasive type of growth, and their malignant nature was proved not only by the destructive character of these local lesions but by the appearance of metastases.

Subsequently Rous and his collaborators Beard and Kidd found that even without interference the malignant change occurred in the domestic rabbit in a high proportion of cases provided the tumors were left to themselves for a certain time. Generally between the fourth and the seventh month there came a change in their appearance, they began to infiltrate the underlying connective tissue of the skin, ulcerated, and eventually metastasized. The transformation set in gradually and often at different sites, so that in animals with a large number of warts it was possible to find 15 or 20 of these simultaneously progressing to cancer. Under the microscope they presented all the characteristic features of squamous cell carcinoma.

The malignant change, common in the domestic rabbit, is a great rarity in the wild cottontail.

The difference in the course of the tumor in the two varieties of rabbit is reflected in wide differences in the behavior of the virus. In papillomas of the cottontail it is so plentiful that it can be obtained in generous amounts even from the cornified masses that detach themselves from the warts, where its high resistance to drying permits it to retain its activity over long periods of time. This it is that underlies the transfer of the disease under natural conditions; in entering their burrows rabbits are apt to sustain abrasions of the skin by scraping against the walls, and thus to inoculate themselves with virus contained in scaly fragments from the papillomas of other rabbits.

In the domestic rabbit, on the contrary, no virus can be found in the papillomas; the animal can be infected with a filtrate but the papillomas that arise cannot be transmitted from one domestic rabbit to another. Its tumors are unquestionably caused by a virus, but one who was unfamiliar with their origin would have not the slightest reason to suspect it.

The presence of virus can be proved, however, by serological methods, for Rous and Kidd have shown that antibodies appear in the blood of the cottontail as the tumors develop. As is always the case in virus infections, these are incapable of getting at virus that has safely reached the cells but are still able to protect the host against reinfection. Precisely the same thing is true of the domestic rabbit. Virucidal antibodies make their appearance in the blood in increasing amounts, keeping pace with the development of the papillomas, so that the virus must perpetuate itself in the tumors. Does it persist also in the carcinomas derived from them?

The answer to this question can be obtained in only one way: inoculating these neoplasms and examining the blood of the hosts for antibodies. Rous and Kidd made this experiment, taking their grafts from a lymph node metastasis to eliminate any error that might have resulted from the presence in a carcinoma of cells from the papilloma in which it developed. The experiment, like all those having to do with squamous cell carcinomas, was laborious, for these tumors are difficult to transplant as every investigator knows only too well, and Rous and his associates had to use a large number of rabbits of a special strain in order to achieve constant results. Yet they succeeded in propagating through 14 generations a squamous cell carcinoma that had originated in a papilloma, and in demonstrating in the blood of all animals bearing it antibodies against the Shope virus that increased progressively in amount as the carcinomas developed.

Direct methods, naturally, were no more successful in disclosing virus in these carcinomas of the domestic rabbit than in its papillomas. The virus existed in masked form and could be detected only by indirect proof. It became important to know, therefore, what happens in the cottontail when papillomas undergo the malignant change. Does the virus persist in the carcinomas as it does in the papillomas?

The difficulty here was that papillomas of the wild rabbit are very seldom transformed into carcinoma. In fact, no such case was known when the problem first presented itself, but a timely paper by Syverton and Berry showed that the change does occur from time to time and a collaborating trapper furnished the desired material. Examination of the several thousand wild rabbits that he provided confirmed the extraordinary frequency of papillomas and the great rarity of malignant transformation, for among all these animals only 6 had carcinomas; in several of the 6 the tumors had metastasized.

No free virus could be found in any of these carcinomas, though in noncancerous papillomas from the same animals it was present in abundance. Furthermore, emulsions of the carcinomas not only held no demonstrable virus but even inactivated virus brought into contact with them; hence they must have contained large amounts of virucidal antibodies.

Thus in the cottontail, as in the domestic rabbit, the malignant transformation goes hand in hand with a disappearance of free virus.

How is all this to be explained?

At first Rous suspected the antibodies. Although some papillomas in the wild rabbit contained generous quantities of virus others in the same animals held very little, and it was noticed that these latter were always deeply fissured and secondarily infected. As capillary fragility is well known to accompany inflammation it was thought that antibodies might easily escape from the blood stream and, accumulating in the damaged tissues, reach and inactivate virus in infected cells as soon as the cell membrane had been injured. The same capillary fragility might be expected in carcinomas, also, because the stroma is always more or less inflamed.

Up to a certain point these suppositions may explain the failure to recover active virus from inflamed or cancerous papillomas, but they do not explain the invariable absence of free virus from the ordinary warts of the domestic rabbit. It seems hardly probable that their capillaries should be abnormally permeable, in the absence of any secondary infection; besides, they are free of demonstrable virus from the very first, when there are no antibodies in the blood.

An interesting observation by Shope introduces an entirely new aspect of the problem. He found that different strains of the papilloma virus show appreciable differences in behavior, and succeeded in isolating one that remained active even in the domestic rabbit. The papillomas that it elicited grew very slowly, and the malignant transformation set in much more rarely than with the usual strains. By inoculating a rabbit with this special strain and with an ordinary strain it was possible to obtain, side by side in the same animal, papillomas from which virus could be liberated and others from which it could not, a proof that antibodies play only a secondary role and that a solution to the problem of free and masked virus must be sought in the behavior of the virus itself. Perhaps in the latter state it is combined with some component of the cell in a union that cannot be dissolved. This is only a hypothesis, certainly, but at the moment it is impossible to say more.

It is especially interesting that virus should be free in papillomas of the cottontail rabbit, yet pass into the masked state as soon as the malignant transformation supervenes. The advent of carcinoma seems to coincide with some fundamental alteration in the virus, and this, together with certain other evidence, led Rous to associate the malignant change with a mutation of the virus.

All this work on the Shope rabbit papilloma has contributed greatly to our knowledge of mammalian virus tumors, but it would be wrong to regard this neoplasm as the only one of its kind and to close this section without even mentioning the virus tumors of man. These are the common warts, the laryngeal papillomas, and the condylomas, or venereal warts.

The old belief that blood from a wart will produce a crop of new ones if spread on the skin has long since been confirmed by accurate clinical observation. Ciuffo, and later Wile and Kingery, have offered incontestable evidence that warts are caused by a filterable virus, and the transmissibility of laryngeal papillomas was accidentally demonstrated by Ullmann; the instrument with which he had just removed one lightly scratched the patient's lip as he was withdrawing it and a few months later warts appeared at this very site.

Later experiments by Dahmann have established the close relationship between laryngeal papillomas and warts of the skin.

Papillomas of the mucous membrane of the genital organs, or venereal warts, were for years attributed to syphilis or gonorrhea, but as it was slowly realized that they may arise in the absence of any venereal disease their autonomous character become more and more evident. The various infections that so often accompany their development are therefore a predisposing factor only. The first experimental demonstration of this was furnished by Waelsch, who inoculated himself subcutaneously with a filtrate from condylomas that had appeared in another physician who was free of syphilis, and some time later saw warts arise at the inoculation site.

Recently Green, Goodlow, Evans, Peyton, and Titrud transplanted a wart from the eyelid of a seventy-one year old man into the anterior chamber of the eye in three monkeys. Epithelial tumors developed simultaneously in all three at the point in the conjunctiva where the inoculating needle had penetrated. For several reasons the authors were inclined to think that these did not come merely from proliferation of the grafts but were actual neoplasms of the conjunctiva itself inaugurated by a virus.

The more or less narrow species specificity characteristic of the viruses has unfortunately prevented repetition of such experiments on a larger scale, but even these few observations are of value because they show that man, too, has his virus tumors. Of course they are not cancers, but neither is the Shope papilloma, though it takes but little to transform its etiological agent into a carcinogenic virus.

When all these isolated facts are put together there is no denying that a long road has been traveled since Borrel first established his virus hypothesis on its pitifully slender basis. The existence of leukemias and of benign and malignant neoplasms, all due to viruses, can no longer be gainsaid and the domain of these lesions, which for many years seemed restricted to birds, has been extended. The Shope papilloma has broken down the barrier arbitrarily erected by adversaries of the infection hypothesis between the malignant avian neoplasms and those of the mammals.

The highly important fact has been established that a tumor may be caused by a virus even though none can be recovered from it by current methods, and it is no longer justifiable to conclude, therefore, that a virus is certainly absent. The hope of success encourages perseverance where only a few years ago no one would have ventured even to try.

One fact of the greatest interest, finally, is the rapidity with which the viruses work. All the other carcinogenic agents so far recognized require a prolonged latent period, and thus appear to be indirect causes only, whereas the viruses seem to act directly. This must inevitably have its weight when we come to assess the relative importance of the factors that are known at present to be concerned in the genesis of cancer.

V

CONCLUSION: ONE KIND OF CANCER OR MANY?

THE four preceding chapters recapitulate the more noteworthy attempts to explain the origin of cancer as they appear in the light of modern experimental research. If there were any wish to remain within the confines of established fact the review would be finished, but it is to be feared that such a course would leave the reader in utter confusion. He could justly accuse the author of having presented him with a mass of unrelated facts without the slightest effort to coördinate them, and of abandoning the subject at the very moment when he expected to hear at last the final word on the problem.

The classical hypotheses all failed in their purpose of furnishing a satisfactory explanation. The work on transplantable tumors provided some interesting information on the *behavior* of cancer but none on its *cause*. Hope then turned to a new method, the initiation of cancer, since it had been the belief for many years that once it became possible to inaugurate malignant growth at will the problem of etiology would be solved. It would be necessary only to analyze minutely all the prevailing experimental conditions, somewhat as a problem in mathematics is solved.

We are sadder and wiser today. We know that malignant growth can be elicited by a variety of processes, that radiant energy, parasites, hereditary factors, chemical compounds, viruses, all lead to the same end, but when it comes to drawing conclusions, to offering a definite opinion on the causes of cancer, we are nonplussed.

We have the uneasy sensation that we know at once too much and too little.

Too much, because instead of one solution we are offered a whole series of them. Suppose for the moment that of all the experimental work we had heard only of that dealing with heredity. We should not hesitate a moment in proclaiming that the problem had been solved. Everything would be clear. Cancer would be linked to hereditary factors and all external influences, acting as does the developer on a photographic image, would but serve to reveal what had already been impressed on the genes.

We should feel equally complacent if we were aware only of the investigations on the carcinogenic hydrocarbons. What could be plainer? Knowing that there are substances of which a fraction of a milligram will elicit cancer regularly and inevitably, knowing that the body can make these from the hormones or the bile acids, we should regard the problem as one simply of biological chemistry. Why trouble to seek further?

Well, because there would still remain the cancer due to heredity, to viruses, to parasites, and to still other factors.

All this leads to the suspicion that the real cause, the innermost mechanism of the malignant change, must lie where all these causes meet. That point, we may be sure, is somewhere in the cell. And it is precisely here that we know too little.

Standing before the cell, we are like one who has been asked to explain the working of an automobile from its external appearance alone. He may proceed after the manner of the physiologist, analyzing what is put into the machine to make it go, and what comes out, but he may not raise the hood. He may ignite or dissolve the whole vehicle to determine its total content of metal and combustible material, but that is all. How can he possibly form any idea of the motor, or of the thousand and one accessories requisite to function? Yet the cell is infinitely more complex, and the derangement that we call cancer is hidden away deep in some inaccessible terra incognita. All hope of acquaintance with what in scientific terms is known as the pathogenic mechanism of cancer must be renounced for the present.

Abandoning speculation on the intrinsic, or final, cause, then, we focus our attention on such extrinsic, or secondary, causes as may be vouchsafed us by experimental research.

These are many, so many, indeed, that we are tempted to draw the astonishing conclusion that cancer is not one single disease, and that instead of saying *cancer* we ought to say *cancers*.

Such a conception has the unquestionable advantage of being in perfect accord with the facts, and those who are timid about leaving the solid ground of reality will be perfectly content because it cannot be refuted by even the most determined argument. Nor can it be denied that to admit a plurality of causes is to contribute to progress. Those who accept or reject heredity *in toto* commit a regrettable error in not distinguishing among the various kinds of cancer. Too long have we used our ignorance of the final cause as an excuse for neglecting to seek out the contributing causes by minute investigation of every case. The factors involved in the genesis of cancer of the stomach and cancer of the breast, for example, are certainly different. It could not be otherwise for epithelium exposed to such dissimilar surroundings and conditions in respect to growth rhythm, sensitivity to hormones, biochemical environment, circulatory states, possibilities of infection, and so on. Of secondary import though they be, these intermediate causes should receive the closest scrutiny, for in this way we can learn to prevent, even though the final cause be the same.

From a practical point of view, therefore, it is quite right that the multiplicity of causes should be emphasized, but the problem changes entirely when examined by the experimentalist in his laboratory. Then the significance of the various etiological factors takes on a totally different aspect. For the clinician, roentgen cancer is caused by X rays, and he knows very well that by taking the necessary precautions he can prevent it. For him the problem is solved. But for the experimentalist the problem is not solved; for him, the X rays may be only a predisposing factor whose carcinogenic activities are subordinated to other conditions.

To the experimentalist the idea that cancer is a whole group of disorders, each with a different cause, is wholly unsatisfactory since no matter how strongly the etiological dissimilarities be emphasized cancer to him is one disease, and one disease only. He sees always the same cellular derangement, marked by exalted proliferation, invasive growth, and above all by the impudent independence that is called autonomy. Whether the malignant cell be found in chicken, rabbit, or man these features are always present, and it is difficult indeed for him to see how there could be so many causes for one and the same disease. Borst expressed this idea perfectly when he said that any hypothesis taking account of only one group of neoplasms, and not applicable to all others, may be rejected at first sight.

Doubts that the real cause is multiple are strengthened by the recollection that the history of cancer is far from unique in this respect. A number of causes have been invoked for other maladies as well, until discovery of the true one put an end to all guesswork. Thus tuberculosis was once attributed to heredity, malnutrition, bad sanitary surroundings, colds, or contact with a tuberculous patient, and to this long list there may be added the industrial causes to which were ascribed the tuberculosis of quarrymen, glass blowers, and so on. Discovery of the tubercle bacillus by Koch reduced the causes to one; it did not eliminate the others, but it did relegate them to a secondary position. For the hygienist the contributing causes still retain all their importance, for it is these that he attacks in his endeavors to stamp out the disease. For the investigator, on the contrary, the multiplicity is a thing of the past and the tubercle bacillus alone the focus of interest.

With cancer, too, it seems difficult to assign equal rank to all the causes suggested by experimental research. There must be some fundamental difference, surely, between the pathogenic activity of parasites that lead to cancer in 5 or 10 per cent of cases, and that of the carcinogenic hydrocarbons that regularly afford 100 per cent of positive results. Nor can like significance be granted to a burn that is followed by a malignant growth after the lapse of 30 years and a virus that accomplishes the same end in 15 days.

One is therefore led to arrange the manifold etiological factors in a graded series, holding one of them to be the principal cause and all the remainder secondary. Naturally this will complicate the problem, for instead of several varieties of cancer, each with a different cause, there will now be but one, with a main cause and a number of accessory causes. It is the operation of these many adjuvants, in all their possible combinations, that produces the neoplasms of apparently different etiology encountered by the clinician and the investigator.

The objection may be raised that there is no point in thus complicating the problem, but daily experience teaches that etiology is almost always a highly complex matter, and the more we learn about a disease the more clearly do we come to understand that the factors coöperating in its production are many and varied.

Let tuberculosis serve once more as an example. Its cause is the bacillus of Koch, and inoculation of a few of these organisms into a guinea pig is enough to determine an inevitable and fatal malady. In man, however, this is not the case. Millions of persons are accidentally inoculated during the course of their lives yet do not become actually tuberculous, for to transform their latent infections into active and progressive disease a number of conditions must be realized; it is here that the accessory causes assume all their importance. Hence we say that in the guinea pig tuberculosis is not conditioned whereas in man it is, and to a rather high degree.

In the light of present knowledge cancer, too, seems a highly conditioned disorder, requiring the concurrence of a number of events. But which among all these is principal?

The factor to which this role shall be given must meet the three following demands:

1. It must be carcinogenic.
2. It must be present in every malignant tumor.

3. Its intervention must be consonant with all other recognized carcinogenic factors and explain their activity.

From this competition radioactivity, parasites, and heredity may be eliminated at once, since obviously they are not concerned in the genesis of every malignant neoplasm. The chemical compounds and the viruses remain.

Invariable presence is theoretically possible for either, but if the chemical compounds be the true cause they must participate in the initiation of virus tumors also. Then it would have to be admitted that of themselves the viruses cannot inaugurate malignant growth, but have to operate indirectly by forming carcinogenic compounds.

This explicitly controverts the known facts. The viruses can and do produce neoplasms, and, furthermore, work much more promptly than the chemicals they would be supposed to elaborate; they can bring about the malignant change in a few days or weeks, whereas the chemical carcinogens all have a much longer latent period.

Thus priority rests with the viruses, but in advancing them to this role we enter the domain of pure speculation. Nevertheless, only two possibilities appear today:

Either we must agree that there are many different kinds of malignant growth, and thus be free to admit as many causes as we wish; or that there is but one malignant process, in which case the virus hypothesis becomes the only logical solution.

Since it is thus, it will be interesting to examine the latter alternative a little more closely, to study the arguments that plead in its favor and those that are arrayed against it.

We shall start by determining whether or not viruses respond to the three requisites just set forth.

As for the first of these, *carcinogenic activity*, discussion is unnecessary. A whole series of viruses is now recognized, and they act much more rapidly than any other carcinogenic agent so far discovered.

The second demands the *constant presence* of a carcinogenic virus in every neoplasm. As a matter of fact, this postulate goes much further, for if viruses be responsible for every single tumor they must of necessity intervene in the genesis of those elicited by chemical compounds. Then, as some carcinogenic hydrocarbons are almost uniformly successful, it would have to be admitted that all animals susceptible to these agents contain viruses for all types of tumors that might conceivably arise under the influence of the carcinogens. There might be a moment's natural hesitation in conceding that viruses can be so widely distributed, but on reflection nothing can be found to oppose the idea. Do not all human beings without exception harbor the colon bacillus and many other microbes in their intestinal tracts? What is possible for microbes ought not be denied to the viruses, the more so because these latter, obligate intracellular parasites that they are, lie sheltered from the reactions that the body sets up against microbes. Nay more, do not the viruses themselves furnish the best example of wide distribution, affecting as they do all among certain kinds of plants and animals?

But here another difficulty presents itself. As the varieties of neoplasia are legion, and each virus elicits in general the same sort of tumor, there would have to be acknowledged not only a wide distribution but an amazing multiplicity of viruses. Well, nature has never been niggardly in such matters, and nothing is more astounding than the prodigious number of varieties included in certain species. Nearly 7,000 are known to take part in putrefaction, so why not allow a much smaller number of cancer viruses? In any case, the total that would be required to inaugurate all the known types of neoplasms may not be so extravagant after all; the propensity of viruses to vary in their cytotropism must not be lost to view. In our own experiments on the viruses of leukemia, as well as in those of Duran-Reynals with the Rous agent, a single virus was seen to give rise to the most diverse neoplastic lesions.

One last question on this subject remains to be answered. If viruses intervene in the genesis of all malignant neoplasms why is it that they cannot invariably be recovered? A partial reply is given by the experiments of Rous with the carcinoma derived from the Shope rabbit papilloma, in which it was shown that a virus actually may be present in a tumor even though it cannot be demonstrated by any means now known. If this masked state result from combination with some constituent of the cell the phenomenon would be apt to affect precisely the carcinogenic viruses, for in order to be cytostimulating a virus must create the smallest possible intracellular disturbance; that is to say, must utilize material that is least needed by the cell on its lawful occasions. In short, it must act virtually like a normal component, if the cell is to survive and react only by excessive multiplication.

But there is still another reason why carcinogenic viruses are so seldom recoverable from malignant tumors. The only available way of demonstrating their presence is the inauguration of a neoplasm with a tumor filtrate, in an animal of the same species. But it is evident that failure by no means proves their absence. Far from it. If it did there is a good chance that most of the vertebrates would long since have perished from the earth. The neoplasms that can be easily transmitted by filtrates correspond to infections that are but lightly conditioned; it is very probable that they are exceptions, and that if cancer in general be caused by viruses they are highly conditioned. Under such circumstances the injection of a tumor filtrate into an animal that is normal and unprepared would have not the slightest chance of success. The virus might be present, but there would be no means of proving it.

There are two procedures that would perhaps better considerably the results so far obtained in experiments of this sort.

The first consists in preparing the animals that are to be injected in such a way as to make their cells receptive to the virus whose presence it is desired to reveal. A start in this direction has already been made by Rous, who employed tarring, and with remarkable success, as we shall see. Other means, too, could be tried; hereditary factors, X rays, hormones, perhaps. The object, in brief, is to imitate natural processes by bringing about the preparatory condition that permits a carcinogenic virus to disclose its presence.

The second method is demonstration of a virus by indirect, or serological, methods. Here, also, some preliminary work has been done. The experiments of Kidd make it very probable that a virus exists in the Brown-Pearce tumor, a carcinoma of the rabbit that can be transplanted by grafts but has never yet been transmitted by a filtrate.

Finally, the relationship of certain carcinogenic viruses to the cells that they have infected may differ fundamentally from the conditions of intracellular parasitism already known, and the mysterious results of Berry and Dedrick with the virus of rabbit myxomatosis suggest entirely new possibilities.

As has already been explained, the myxoma virus and the fibroma virus show the phenomenon of cross immunity, and may therefore be thought of as closely related. Berry and Dedrick inoculated rabbits with a mixture of active fibroma virus and myxoma virus that had been inactivated by exposure to a temperature of 60° or 75°C. for half an hour. And then, something very curious happened. Because of its contact with the living fibroma virus the myxoma virus, assumed to be dead, recovered its activity and the animals died of myxomatosis. The virus thus restored to life in these rabbits was highly virulent, and could easily be transmitted once more in series. As these experiments have been confirmed in several laboratories, according to Shope, there can be no doubt as to the accuracy of the observation.

What must have taken place was a sort of vital induction. Perhaps a virus can transmit to an inert substance, as we may well suppose a virus inactivated by heat to be, a capacity to multiply inside the cell; and if an inactivated virus can thus be resurrected, and incited to autonomous growth, what stands in the way of imagining that a like stimulus may sometimes be felt by normal cell components also, at the instigation of an invading virus?

Carcinogenic activity would then present a wholly different front. A virus, entirely harmless in itself, perhaps, would transfer the spark to certain molecular groups in a cell, which thenceforth could multiply autonomously and behave as a virus, though actually still a part of the cell. Thrown off balance by the disordered and incessant growth of one of its own constituents, the cell, in its turn, would be constantly driven to divide without respect to the needs of the body. And this, after all, is the characteristic feature of malignant growth. It would not be surprising if such a tumor could not be transmitted with filtrates, for in killing its cells one would have killed at the same time the factors responsible for their exaggerated multiplication.

We come now to the third and last postulate, according to which the cause chosen as intrinsic must be *compatible with all others* recognized as carcinogenic. And here we shall consider the viruses in their relation with neoplasms ascribed to parasites, to chemical agents, and to heredity.

VIRUSES AND NEOPLASMS ASCRIBED TO PARASITES

As the carcinogenic activity of parasites is always inconstant, being exerted in only a small proportion of cases, the parasite itself does not seem to be the sole cause. Hence Borrel was led to suspect the intervention of another factor, and to suggest that a parasite can induce malignant growth only when it carries a virus with which it can infect susceptible cells as it makes its way through the tissues. Its role, therefore, would be simply that of an inoculator.

Acting on this belief, he prophesied that when virus was absent there would be negative experiments with parasites which, like *Gongylonema neoplasticum*, are reputed to be carcinogenic, and his prediction was fully realized as we have already seen. Bullock and Curtis, on the other hand, convinced that the parasite itself would be able to initiate a malignant tumor provided the constitution of the host were favorable, attributed the irregularity of their results to hereditary influences and mutation.

The facts, on the whole, favor Borrel's view. The participation of hereditary factors is possible, probable even; but were they the sole cause positive results should have been indiscriminately and equally divided among all experiments with animals of mixed stock. Actually, cancer appeared in a rather high proportion of the animals in some series, as in the experiments of Fibiger, and not at all in others, like those of Passey.

Moreover, the dissemination of virus diseases by parasites is no purely imaginative occurrence but an actual fact, as the recent experiments of Shope with swine influenza demonstrate. The virus of this disease may enter the body of a nematode belonging to the Strongylus group that often infests the bronchi in swine. The eggs reach the mouth in the bronchial secretions, are swallowed, and finally eliminated with the feces. They are then eaten by earthworms, in whose organisms the eggs develop as far as the larval stage and persist as such, sometimes over a long period, until the worm is eaten by a pig. Here the larvae penetrate the walls of the digestive tract, to be carried by the blood stream to the bronchi where they are transformed into adult worms. The virus may retain its activity throughout this whole cycle, for Shope was able to transmit the disease with parasites that had been in the larval stage for as long as two years.

These observations provide information of the greatest interest. In the first place, they display parasites in the role assigned them by Borrel: vectors for a virus. The role is not entirely neutral, however. The parasite does not carry the virus as a simple pollution, but offers the possibility of retaining its pathogenic properties for years, though under ordinary circumstances this virus can be preserved in active condition hardly more than two months. Thus the parasite actually plays toward it the part of an intermediate host.

Secondly, the virus exists in a masked state within the body of the parasite, as the Shope virus does in papillomas of the domestic rabbit.

In the face of such facts as these it would be difficult to hold the virus hypothesis incompatible in any way with the production of malignant tumors by parasites. On the contrary, their role as carriers and intermediate hosts may of itself explain any irregularities in the development of neoplasms ascribed to them.

Indeed, the role of parasites in the etiology of cancer is likely from now on to assume greater importance than would have been thought possible only a few years ago. It seems curious that most geneticists, though they investigate so conscientiously the mammary carcinomas of the mouse, still continue to neglect *Muspicea borreli,* the nematode that Borrel encountered with such frequency in association with these neoplasms. Again, we are completely ignorant of the way in which the virus tumors and leukemias of birds are transmitted under natural conditions; perhaps the situation is something like that obtaining for swine influenza, and parasites thought to be harmless are actually the carriers of viruses that cause them.

VIRUSES AND TUMORS ASCRIBED TO CHEMICAL AGENTS

THE idea that a virus may be responsible for neoplasms that follow the application of carcinogenic compounds seems at first sight hardly plausible, and has been called even absurd. But for those who believe all malignant growth to be a single process it is a logical necessity, and experimental research has already brought forward some singularly pertinent facts.

The tar cancer that develops on the rabbit's ear after 5 or 6 months of painting grows slowly, shows almost no aggressive tendency, and is apt to recede and disappear spontaneously, as Leroux and Simard, together with many others, have emphasized.

In a series of experiments carried out by Rous and Kidd rabbits were painted with tar for 2 or 3 months, and at the first appearance of the ordinary discrete, slowly growing papillomas were given a large dose of a filtrate of the Shope papilloma by intravenous injection. In unpainted control rabbits this had no effect, for the virus evidently encountered no receptive cells. But in the tarred animals the papillomas already present began to grow rapidly after 15 to 20 days, and new tumors even arose throughout the tarred areas. These rapidly became fleshy masses, and within a short time showed their malignant nature by invading the underlying tissues until they had penetrated to the opposite side of the ear, and by finally metastasizing. This was no chance occurrence, for it could be reproduced every time the experiment was repeated, and Lacassagne and Nyka reported a similar outcome when benzpyrene was substituted for tar.

Thus the Shope virus, introduced into a rabbit whose epidermal cells are intact, is unable to invade them, but it can seize upon the epidermis when this has been prepared by a carcinogen, and bring about the malignant change after a much shorter interval than the carcinogen alone would require.

These observations prove that carcinogens can prepare cells for the advent of carcinogenic viruses. Furthermore, a rapid development and high malignancy distinguish cancers thus produced from those elicited with tar or benzpyrene alone.

The experiments just mentioned are supplemented by the investigations of Andrewes, Ahlström, Foulds, and Gye. The virus of the Shope rabbit fibroma, injected under the skin of the domestic variety, produces connective tissue growths at the inoculation site that regress after a few weeks of proliferation. Somewhat as in the experiments of Rous and Kidd, rabbits were prepared by the intramuscular injection of tar, and fibroma virus was administered intravenously later. The tissues bordering on the tar deposits gave rise to fibromas that grew with unusual rapidity, one of which proved to be frankly sarcomatous.

On the other hand, no agent reacting upon hyperplastic tissues in the mouse as do the Shope papilloma and fibroma viruses in the rabbit could be found by Woglom in mouse sarcoma 37, though in various experiments throughout the world this growth has often seemed just on the point of declaring a viral origin.

Finally, it may be observed that the constantly increasing number of carcinogenic agents is leading the chemical hypothesis into a blind alley. It is not impossible to imagine that the carcinogenic hydrocarbons and the aromatic amines may initiate malignant growth in a more or less direct manner, but when it is added that hydrochloric acid, and sugar too, can achieve this result, the situation becomes wholly incomprehensible. Some day the chemists themselves, though now so generally in opposition to the virus hypothesis, will have to enlist its aid as malignant tumors are produced with greater frequency by substances that are even more bland. And if the intervention of other factors should prove necessary to explain some of the malignant growths that follow the application of chemical compounds, why stop there? Why not include them all? Thanks to experimental research the participation of viruses in the production of these neoplasms has lost much of its improbability. In any case, the virus hypothesis need no longer be thought incompatible with established ideas on the inauguration of tumors with chemicals.

VIRUSES AND TUMORS ASCRIBED TO HEREDITY

In examining selectively bred strains of mice in which cancer appears with almost disconcerting regularity, in perceiving how crosses arranged with respect to pedigree may cause certain tumors to come or go at the will of the investigator, one asks not unnaturally what part a virus could possibly take in this process. All seems to be so competently managed by heredity that the intrusion of an external influence looks almost inconceivable. It should not be forgotten, however, that the role of heredity once appeared equally well established for tuberculosis, yet no one would now deny the infectious nature of this disease.

As a matter of fact, the infection hypothesis does not run counter to what is known of heredity.

Both microbes and viruses exhibit subtleties in their aggressions that may be surprising but that exist nevertheless.

Of this tuberculosis offers a striking example. Physicians of a bygone day attributed the chief role to heredity, but with the discovery of the tubercle bacillus, and of the way in which it enters the body, the importance of heredity was lost to view. Now, however, heredity is regaining its former position little by little, and investigations of the past few years have restored its former dignity to a conception that never would have been neglected had it not been for the effort to prove an incompatibility between heredity and infection. Here, again, monochorial twins are a fertile field for investigation, and Kallman and Reisner have recently published some observations that bear a singular resemblance to what has been described on preceding pages for cancer.

What is true for tuberculosis applies to many other infections as well, and experimental medicine is finding it more and more necessary to take heredity into account.

Susceptibility to virus infections also seems to be frequently associated with hereditary characters, and if the virus of St. Louis encephalitis, for example, strikes with perfect selectivity at the mice of some strains why deny the same property to certain carcinogenic viruses?

But the role of the viruses in cancerous heredity may be explained in still another way.

For some time now investigators like Little, Korteweg, MacDowell and Richter, and Lynch have been recording facts that do not square with the general conception of chromosomal heredity. Thus differences in the results of crosses between mice of cancer and noncancer strains, according to whether the male or the female belonged to the susceptible strain, would hardly be expected on a theoretical basis. Actually, however, the female influence was always found predominant, so definitely so, indeed, that Little was led to reject wholly the mendelian nature of heredity for cancer of the mamma in mice.

But many years earlier it had occurred to Borrel that the assumed hereditary transmission of susceptibility to mammary carcinoma in this species might be connected with the passage of a carcinogenic virus from mother to offspring by way of parasites or of the milk. To explore this possibility he exchanged newborn mice from mothers of cancer and noncancer strains, with results that appear not to have belied his suspicion, though it is difficult to assess his results because his strains were not really inbred.

The investigation has been resumed by Bittner, however, with unimpeachable material, and has borne fruit in the shape of a discovery whose scope cannot yet be foreseen.

When newborn mice from a cancer strain were allowed to suckle a mother from a noncancer strain the incidence of mammary carcinoma among them, when they reached maturity, decreased in a surprising manner. But what would be the outcome of a converse experiment? Can the incidence be increased, in strains where cancer is rare or absent, by putting the young to nurse on mothers from high cancer strains? Many authors agree that it can, and Andervont, for example, describes experiments in which the incidence was lowered from 100 per cent to 50 per cent, or raised from 0 per cent to 71 per cent, by appropriate foster nursing. The latter result is not invariably realized, but one important fact is to be noted; a mouse receiving this "milk influence," which favors the development of cancer, may transmit it by means of her milk even though she herself never fall victim to the disease.

Something of the highest significance must pass over with the milk, and the idea comes naturally to mind that it may be a virus. Bittner and many others suspect this to be the case, but unfortunately it has not yet been proved. Recent investigations seem to indicate that the milk influence is of a much more general nature, and affects the whole organism. The science of genetics may be collapsing before our eyes.

But however this may be, the conclusion may fairly be drawn that the virus hypothesis is not in conflict with what is known of the relations between heredity and cancer, and it has now been shown to satisfy all three of our postulates.

Some objections, however, still remain to be discussed.

It is often said that the virus hypothesis cannot be accepted because cancer is not contagious, but this reasoning is based on a misconception; an infectious disease is not necessarily contagious in the ordinary sense of the word. *Herpes labialis* (fever blister) and *herpes zoster* (shingles), both due to viruses and therefore both infectious diseases, are not contagious, nor are the leukemias and filterable sarcomas of the fowl that are maintained in laboratories, though each bird affected carries enough virus to infect millions of others.

The contagiousness of an infection depends upon the transmissibility of the causative agent and the receptivity of the organism that it encounters. If both be at a maximum the infection spreads without hindrance and soon acquires the proportions of an epidemic. If one be lacking the thread is broken and contagion does not occur.

Typhus fever is one of the most murderous infections with which the human race is cursed, and whole populations have been wiped out by it. Yet see upon what a little thing its transmission depends. A louse! A typhus patient without lice is no more capable of transmitting the disease than a cancer patient his.

Thus contagiousness may be abolished by the absence of a specific carrier, and the same result may follow when the subject attacked is not susceptible. Receptivity toward poliomyelitis, for example, is not apt to be high; furthermore, the disease may occur in the form of sporadic cases and all attempts to trace the route taken by the virus in reaching these patients may fail. Imagine, now, the existence of a virus much more widely distributed but also much more highly conditioned, and we should have that of herpes or of cancer. For so far as can be known at present the development of cancer requires the coöperation of a large number of factors; and lack of contagiousness is the sign of a highly conditioned infection.

Most objections raised against the virus hypothesis reveal an imperfect knowledge of the rationale of infection, for there is still often encountered the outmoded notion that microbes and viruses attack indiscriminately, eliciting their diseases immediately and inevitably.

As an instance of this, it is asserted that constant presence and wide diffusion of carcinogenic viruses would be incompatible with the occurrence of cancer at certain characteristic periods of life. But it must not be forgotten that infections may be conditioned by age, by the state of the endocrine glands, and by a whole series of other factors. Thus ringworm of the scalp is seen only in children and disappears promptly at puberty, but when atrophy of the testes occurs by some mischance in the adult it creates anew a favorable soil and the disease reappears. No chemist has ever discovered the changes that take place in the hair follicles under the influence of puberty. The fungus of ringworm is more knowing.

Why may not the activity of carcinogenic viruses be similarly associated with changes occurring in the body during the various periods of life?

In the fact that cancer can be elicited with tar some see conclusive proof against the intervention of an infectious agent, since tar is strongly antiseptic. But who ever suggested that the virus of cancer is present in tar? In any case, Rous and Kidd have clearly shown that tarring not only does not prevent the infection of cells by the Shope virus but, on the contrary, favors it.

A criticism that appears at first sight to be more damaging is that of F. C. Wood: As malignant cells can be killed with doses of X ray much smaller than those required to destroy viruses, it should be possible to kill the cells of a neoplasm without eradicating a hypothetical virus; yet tumors in which the cells have been killed by X rays cannot be transmitted. The objection does not hold, however, for growths in which a free virus has been found, since in the experiments of Peacock, described on a preceding page, chicken sarcoma was completely destroyed by radiation yet the virus remained active and subsequently induced other sarcomas.

As for the tumors from which virus cannot be recovered, even though it were not annulled there is no way known of demonstrating its presence. Moreover, the resistance of viruses to chemical and physical agents varies greatly according to their condition at the moment, as may be so clearly seen in the bacteriophages.

These, like all the other viruses, are very sensitive to heat, and prolonged exposure to 56°C. kills them almost without exception. On the other hand, some microbes are able to transform themselves into inactive forms called spores, which are highly resistant to heat; even a long immersion in boiling water does not destroy them, and to kill them they must be exposed to temperatures above 120°C. If such microbes are infected by a bacteriophage this may pass into the spores, which then confer upon it the resistance to heat and other physical agents that they themselves enjoy, the bacteriophage integrating itself with the spore as though actually a part of it. What is true of increased resistance should be true also of diminished resistance, and would be much easier to understand. In other words, there is nothing opposed to the idea that in certain phases of their life cycle the viruses share the sensitivity of the cells that they infect.

Their response to X rays would be more comprehensible if they were known to act indirectly, by setting up an induced autonomy in certain components of the cell, as suggested on a preceding page. In such a case these constituents, responsible for the malignant change, would naturally share the sensitivity of the cell to radiation.

The remorseless nature of cancer is occasionally offered as an argument against the participation of a virus in its etiology. If malignant tumors really are caused by an external agent, the argument runs, they should occasionally disappear of themselves, for there is not a microbic disease, no matter how formidable, that does not show a more or less appreciable percentage of spontaneous recoveries. In the case of cancer, spontaneous cure is so rare that every single case is published, surrounded and supported with every possible guarantee that the neoplasm actually was malignant.

Everyone will admit, however, that it is difficult to estimate the frequency of spontaneous cure because cancer is generally not recognized until it has reached an advanced stage. It is entirely possible that many malignant growths disappear in their initial stages, leaving no trace behind. This, of course, is the purest speculation. But even admitting that cancer never disappears spontaneously, that is no reason for rejecting the virus hypothesis. Sight should never be lost of the fundamental differences, from the standpoint of possible cure, between the diseases caused by microbes and those brought about by the viruses.

As a general rule microbes invade the tissue spaces and the blood stream, where they are exposed to the concerted antagonistic action of phagocytes, humoral antibodies, and chemotherapeutic agents. This is not true of the viruses. Concealed within the cells, they enjoy perfect protection against all attack, and do not become vulnerable until they have destroyed the cells that harbor them. The virus of cancer knows better than to do so, and it is this that gives the disease its implacable character.

Another objection urged against the virus hypothesis is the remarkable stability characterizing the various strains of transplantable neoplasms. Mouse tumors are still growing today that have been transplanted continuously for 30 years, without the least change having taken place in their cells. This is more than 10 times the life span of the mouse; how is it possible for any virus to retain its individuality over such a long period of time?

Those who put the question forget that a virus has no need to change its nature, and that 30 years in the life of a species are as but a day. The rabies virus now used in most of the Pasteur Institutes throughout the world is the very strain that was isolated when the treatment was introduced 60 years ago, yet no one seems surprised to find it still active. Then why not assume equal stability for a cancer virus?

Some investigators have considered the virus hypothesis inconsonant with the fact that malignant tumors can be produced experimentally at sites where they never occur spontaneously; in the skin of the rabbit or the mouse, for example. The reply could have been made that the laboratory elicits diseases every day that do not appear under natural conditions, yet are due to infectious agents nevertheless. Actually, no answer is required, for the objection is already obsolete; spontaneous neoplasms of the skin in the rabbit are now known, and their cause is a virus. As for the mouse, a number of spontaneous skin tumors are on record, though so far no attempt has been made to transmit such a growth with a filtrate.

There seems to be a desire to limit the number of viruses, and to admit their existence only at sites where spontaneous tumors are known to arise, a conception that loses all sight of the prodigious multiplicity of microbes. This is freely recognized, for the culture tube and the microscope have convinced us that the microbes inhabiting our skin and mucous membranes can be counted in their millions and thousand millions. Yet the invisible agents of disease we wish to restrict in quantity and in kind, and merely because their presence is disclosed only by the mischief that they do. In truth there is every chance that as to both number and variety the viruses far outstrip anything that we can imagine, and who would venture to assert that none among them are capable of transforming mouse epidermis into carcinoma? There may be hundreds such; the important thing is to find them.

All in all, then, the virus hypothesis contains nothing repellent to the mind, nothing in flagrant contradiction with facts already established. On the contrary, it explains much that otherwise would be entirely incomprehensible.

We need only pass in review some of the facts mentioned in our discussion of the various hypotheses to see that all can be satisfactorily accounted for by the virus hypothesis.

Think for a moment of the proliferative lesions that so often precede by years, or often decades, the appearance of a malignant tumor: rectal polyps, papillomas of the bladder or larynx, Bowen's disease, certain forms of Paget's disease, the follicular psorospermosis of Darrier, and many more. In all these conditions abnormal cells are found that even then may exhibit the cytological characteristics of cancer; they are veritable "cancers in the cradle." Is not all this reminiscent of cells infected with a virus, like those of the Shope papilloma, that live in precarious equilibrium until the day when all the necessary conditions have been fulfilled and the virus itself, or the cell constituents that it has induced thereto, begin their unbridled multiplication and launch the cell on its mad career of malignancy?

The more closely the problem of neoplasia is studied the clearer does it grow that the malignant tumors are but an arbitrary subdivision of a large group containing all the forms of abnormal growth that Galen assembled under the term "tumors contrary to nature." The embryonal neoplasms fully prove this, for among them may be found all types of morbid proliferation and all possible transitions from one to the other. Well, a similar gamut, from the benign fibroma up to the most malignant of neoplasms, is encountered among the virus tumors also.

The only serious objection to be brought against the virus hypothesis at the present time is that it remains unproved. For this reason, and despite the progress of the past few years, most students of cancer prudently elect to support a less graphic conception, one not so exposed to criticism, the hypothesis of somatic mutation in short. This has already been briefly discussed in Chapter III, where it was explained that the term mutation implies an acquisition of new characteristics. A mutation appears suddenly, persists without alteration, and is transmitted indefinitely to descendants of the affected cell. In almost all cases the process involves the sex cells, creating within a species those innumerable varieties that have been so intensively studied for many years by breeders of plants and animals.

Modern genetic research has contributed two discoveries of the highest importance. First, mutations can be made to occur more frequently by exposing germinal cells to radiant energy in any of its forms, such as heat, X rays, and so on, or to certain chemical or mechanical influences. Secondly, mutations thus produced do not differ qualitatively from those occurring naturally; it is only that they are increased in number. In the strings of genes making up the chromosomes there must be weak places predisposed to these mishaps so that, whether spontaneous or provoked, they occur at predestined spots just as a chain parts at its weakest link.

It is tempting to think of the malignant change as a mutation affecting not a sex cell but any cell in the body; in other words, to refer it to somatic mutation. And, indeed, this hypothesis, developed principally by Boveri, Whitman, Bauer, Lockhart-Mummery, Ludford, L. C. Strong, and Sutton, does enjoy high favor, being for most students of cancer, at the moment anyway, the only satisfactory solution and almost a logical postulate.

It is obvious that somatic mutation explains very neatly the irrevocable character of the malignant change, and that the chromosomal irregularities that are one of the salient features of the cancer cell almost automatically suggest some disturbance of these bodies. Furthermore, two arguments add considerable force to the hypothesis. The multiplicity of etiological factors in cancer, stumbling block for so many hypotheses, accords perfectly with that of mutation, for mutations can be brought about by the most varied causes. Again, influences that produce them, such as radiant energy, are in the very front rank of the carcinogenic agents.

It must be confessed that at first sight the hypothesis seems alluring, but upon closer examination serious objections begin to arise.

In the first place, somatic mutations, found principally among the plants and the insects, are exceptionally rare in mammals, and those few that are known invariably affect secondary characters like pigmentation; they are never associated with such a radical change as the malignant transformation of a cell.

Secondly, one of the fundamental attributes of a mutation is sudden appearance. Malignant neoplasms, on the contrary, generally do not arise until after long-continued cellular derangement, and the only ones that by their abrupt development would justify the mutation hypothesis are the virus tumors.

In the third place, the cytological changes preceding the outbreak of most malignant neoplasms may require a number of years for their evolution. At what moment in the process shall we place the mutation? If at the end, what was the nature of the preceding stages? If at the begining, not one but a whole series of successive mutations would have to be acknowledged. And here we fall into absurdity.

Fourth, it has already been explained that there is no qualitative difference between spontaneous and induced mutations. If cancer be the result of a mutation the effect of the carcinogens would be merely to augment the frequency of a phenomenon that might occur spontaneously in any tissue whatsoever. The law of probability should then enable us to assign to every tissue an incidence of spontaneous tumors that would depend above all upon the frequency with which mitosis takes place in it. But all that is known of cancer at present opposes such a supposition. Save for the Shope papilloma, spontaneous cancer of the skin is almost unknown in the mouse and the rabbit, yet this tissue readily undergoes malignant change when carcinogenic agents are applied to it.

Finally, the most serious objection against the mutation hypothesis is the existence of the virus tumors themselves and the fact that the viruses can start the malignant change immediately, so to speak, or at least much more rapidly than any other agent. To this must be added the fact that nuclear abnormalities, to which adherents of the mutation hypothesis attach so much importance, occur also in virus tumors; and it may be remarked in passing that these have never been shown to be primary. They might be secondary. Thus, for example, the achromatic spindle, those radiating threads in which the chromosomes are suspended during cell division, is derived wholly from the cell body, and Ludford points out that anomalies in it cause unequal separation of the chromosomes with asymmetrical mitoses as a consequence. Even though a virus never penetrated the nucleus, therefore, it is readily conceivable that the disturbance resulting from its presence in the cell body could produce nuclear irregularities entirely comparable with those seen in malignant cells.

In the face of all these difficulties the attempt has been made to save the mutation hypothesis by making the viruses themselves the cause of mutation. Then, however, the hypothesis would lose all significance, for instead of saying "malignant transformation" one would merely say "malignant mutation," and be no further forward. But this is only playing with words. The virus tumors can be explained perfectly without recourse to mutation, for the presence of intracellular parasites, or of cell components that have become autonomous, can have but one of two consequences: cell death, or cell multiplication without respect to the needs of the body.

Confronted by the virus hypothesis, that of somatic mutation does not withstand critical examination. To give it the preference is arbitrarily to replace a fact demonstrated for a whole group of neoplasms by a purely speculative idea that adds nothing to what is already known and whose application to the cancer problem is justified by no serious argument.

Arrived now at the end of our journey, we have to confess that the problem of cancer has not been solved, though highly significant facts accumulated during the past few years suggest that it is not insoluble. Alone among the various hypotheses that of the viruses seems to have a real chance of leading to the goal. Only this, whether in its classic form or in the form of induced autonomy, can explain satisfactorily the chief characteristic of the true neoplasms: Autonomy.

To those who may be inclined to reproach the author for a too enthusiastic partisanship he would reply that it is never ill judged to be guided by a hypothesis so long as it does no violence to the known facts, and that the best proof of value is the amount of research stimulated. Submitted to these tests, the virus hypothesis has nothing to fear.

BIBLIOGRAPHY

I. WHY SHOULD CANCER INTEREST US?

BEHAN, R. J. Cancer: With Special Reference to Cancer of the Breast. St. Louis, C. V. Mosby Company, 1938.

BERGER, L., and OBERLING, C. Unpublished observations.

DUBLIN, L. I. Oral communication.

DUFFIELD, T. J., and DI MARIO, M. Cancer Mortality in New York City: 1901 to 1938. *Cancer Research*, 1, 413, 1941.

NICOLLE, C. Biologie de l'invention. Paris, Alcan.

ROUSSY, G. Le Cancer. Nouveau Traité de Médecine, fasc. V, t. 2. 2d ed. Paris, Masson et Cie., 1929.

SCHERESCHEWSKY, J. W. The Course of Cancer Mortality in the Ten Original Registration States for the 21-Year Period, 1900–1920. *U.S. Pub. Health Bull.*, No. 155, 1925.

II. THE DEVELOPMENT OF KNOWLEDGE ON THE NATURE OF CANCER

BARD, L. Cited by Wolff, p. 431.

BICHAT, M. F. X. Anatomie générale. Paris, 1821. Cited by Wolff, p. 89.

COLLARD, R. Mémoire sur les caractères du Cancer. *Bull. Soc. anat.*, 1828. Cited by Wolff, p. 127.

DESCARTES, R. Cited by Wolff, p. 58.

DUMAS. Cited by Klein.

EWING, J. Neoplastic Diseases: A Treatise on Tumors. 4th ed. Philadelphia and London, W. B. Saunders Company, 1940.

GALEN. Cited by Wolff, p. 11.

GLUGE, G. Recherches microscopiques sur le fluide contenu dans les cancers encephaloides. *Compt. rend. Acad. Sci.*, 4, 1837.

HIPPOCRATES. Cited by Wolff, p. 4.

HOOKE, R. Mikrographia, or some physiological Descriptions on minute Bodies by magnifying Glasses. London, 1665. Cited by Wilson, p. 22.

KLEIN, M. Histoire des origines de la théorie cellulaire. No. 3, Exposé histoire philosophies et sciences. Paris, Hermann et Cie., 1937.

LAËNNEC, R. T. H. Cited by Wolff, p. 91.

LEBERT, H. Traité pratique des maladies cancéreuses et des affections curables confondues avec le Cancer. Paris, 1851.

LEYDIG, F. Cited by Klein.

MASSON, P. Les tumeurs. In Traité de Médicine, Ribadeau-Dumas, Sergent Babonneix. Paris, Maloine, 1923.

MÉNÉTRIER, P. E. Nouveau Traité de Médecine. Cancer, t. 13. 2d ed. Paris, Ballière.

MÜLLER, J. Ueber den feineren Bau und die Formen der krankhaften Geschwülste. Berlin, Reimer, 1838.

RASPAIL. Cited by Wolff, p. 126.

ROUSSY, G. Le Cancer. Nouveau Traité de Médecine, fasc. V, t. 2. 2d ed. Paris, Masson et Cie., 1929.

SCHLEIDEN, M. J. Cited by Woglom, p. 3.

SCHWANN, T. Mikroskopische Untersuchungen über die Uebereinstimmung in der Struktur und dem Wachstum der Thiere und Pflanzen. Berlin, Reimer, 1839.

VAN LEEUWENHOEK, A. Secrets of Nature. 1695.

VIRCHOW, R. Die krankhaften Geschwülste. Berlin, 1863.

Wilson, E. B. The Cell in Development and Heredity. New York, The Macmillan Company, 1925.

Woglom, W. H. The Study of Experimental Cancer: A Review. New York, Columbia University Press, 1913.

Wolff, J. Die Lehre von der Krebskrankheit von den Ältesten Zeiten bis zur Gegenwart. I. Teil. Jena, Fischer, 1907.

III. THREE HYPOTHESES

Billroth, T. Cited by Wolff, *passim.*

Borrel, A. Le problème du cancer. *Bull. Inst. Pasteur,* 5, 497, 545, 593, 641, 1907.

——— Epithélioses infectieuses et épithéliomas. *Ann. Inst. Pasteur,* 17, 112, 1903.

Boveri, T. The Origin of Malignant Tumors. Baltimore, Williams and Wilkins Company, 1929. English translation by Marcella Boveri.

Broussais, F. J. V. Cited by Wolff, p. 96.

Cohnheim, J. Congenitales, quergestreiftes Muskelsarkom der Nieren. *Virchows Arch.,* 65, 64, 1875.

——— Vorlesungen über allgemeine Pathologie. Berlin, 1877.

Darier, M. J. Cited by Wolff, pp. 561 ff.

des Ligneris, M. J. A. Precancer and Carcinogenesis. *American J. Cancer,* 40, 1, 1940.

Doyen, E. L. Etiologie et traitement du cancer. Paris, 1904.

Durante. Cited by Wolff, p. 351.

Ewing, J. Neoplastic Diseases: A Treatise on Tumors. 4th ed. Philadelphia and London, W. B. Saunders Company, 1940.

Feinberg, L. Das Gewebe und die Ursache der Krebsgeschwülste. Berlin, 1903. Cited by Wolff, pp. 651 ff.

Fischer-Wasels, B. Allgemeine Geschwulstlehre. Handbuch der normalen und pathologischen Physiologie. Berlin, Springer, 1926.

Hallion, L. Cited by Ménétrier.

Lewin, C. Die Ätiologie der bösartigen Geschwülste. Berlin, Springer, 1928.

Lobstein, J. F. D. Traité d'Anatomie pathologique. Paris, 1829. Cited by Wolff, pp. 100, 340.

Lumière, A. Le cancer, maladie des cicatrices. Paris, Masson et Cie., 1929.

——— Le cancer est-il contagieux? *Ann. d'Hygiene Publique, Industrielle et Sociale,* n.s., 7, 88, 1929.

——— and Mme. Montoloy. Sur la flore microbienne des tumeurs malignes. *Bull. Acad. Méd., Paris,* 97, 767, 1927.

——— and Vigne, P. Existe-t-il des maisons à cancer? *Bull. Acad. Méd.,* Paris, 108, 1288, 1932.

——— ——— Statistiques et maisons à cancer. *Bull. Acad. Méd.,* Paris, 109, 280, 1933.

Masson, P. Les tumeurs. In Traité de Médecine, Ribadeau-Dumas, Sergent Babonneix. Paris, Maloine, 1923.

Ménétrier, P. E. Nouveau Traité de Médecine. Cancer, t. 13. 2d ed. Paris, Ballière.

Müller, J. Ueber den feineren Bau und die Formen der krankhaften Geschwülste. Berlin, Reimer, 1938.

Oberling, C. A propos des glioses meningées (gliose méningoencéphalique) des centres nerveux et du nerf optique. *Rev. canadienne de Biol.,* 2, 120, 1943.

——— Guérin, M., and Zehnder, M. A propos de l'action du jus de tomate injecté dans les tissus. *Bull. Assn. Française pour l'Etude du Cancer,* 22, 401, 1933.

Paget, J. Cited by Ewing.

Rappin, G. Sur le microbe du carcinome. *Compt. rend. Acad. Sci.,* Paris, 198, 1460, 1934.

Récamier, J. C. A. Recherches sur le Traitement du Cancer, etc. Paris, 1829.

Remak, R. Cited by Ewing.

Ribbert, H. Das Karzinom des Menschen. Cohen, Bonn, 1911.
——— Geschwulstlehre. 2d ed. Cohen, Bonn, 1914.
Sawtschenko, J. Weitere Untersuchungen über schmarotzende Sporozoen in den Krebsgeschwülsten. Zentralbl. f. Bakteriol., 12, 17, 1892. Cited by Wolff, p. 635.
Scheurlen Die Aetiologie des Carcinoms. *Berliner klin. Wchnschr.* 24, 935, 1887. Cited by Wolff, p. 546.
Smith, E. F. Studies on the Crown Gall of Plants. Its Relation to Human Cancer. *J. Cancer Research*, 1, 231, 1916.
Unna, P. G. Histopathology of the Diseases of the Skin. English translation by Norman Walker. New York, Macmillan & Company, 1896.
Virchow, R. Cited by Woglom, p. 4.
Wells, H. Gideon. Occurrence and Significance of Congenital Malignant Neoplasms. *Arch. Pathol.*, 30, 535, 1940.
Woglom, W. H. The Study of Experimental Cancer: A Review. New York, Columbia University Press, 1913.
Wolff, J. Die Lehre von der Krebskrankheit von den Ältesten Zeiten bis zur Gegenwart. I. Teil. Jena, G. Fischer, 1907.

IV. EXPERIMENTAL CANCER

THE TRANSPLANTABLE TUMOR

Apolant, H. Ueber die Einwirkung von Radiumstrahlen auf das Karzinom der Mäuse. *Deutsche med. Wchnschr.*, 30, 454, 1904.
Aschoff, L. Cited by Hirschfeld.
Bashford, E. F. The Behaviour of Tumour-Cells During Propagation. Fourth Scientific Report, Imperial Cancer Research Fund. London, Taylor and Francis, 1911.
——— and Murray, J. A. Scientific Reports, Imperial Cancer Research Fund. London, Taylor & Francis, 1904, 1905, 1908.
——— ——— and Cramer, W. Einige Ergebnisse der experimentellen Krebsforschung. *Berliner klin. Wchnschr.*, 42, 1433, 1905.
Besredka, A., Magat, J., Laval, P., and Besnard, P. L'Epithélioma Intracutané du Lapin et son pouvoir immunisant. *Ann. Inst. Pasteur*, 56, 125, 1936.
Biette. Cited by Woglom, p. 43.
Bischoff, F., and Long, M. L. The Relation of the Vitamin B Complex to Tumor Growth. *American J. Cancer*, 37, 54, 1939.
Bonne, C. Fréquénce des métastases pulmonaires dans les cas de tumeurs greffées dans la queue de la souris. *Compt. rend. Soc. Biol.*, 93, 312, 1925.
Borrel, A. Epithélioses infectieuses et Epithéliomas. *Ann. Inst. Pasteur*, 17, 81, 112, 1903.
——— Le problème étiologique du Cancer. *Ztschr. f. Krebsforsch.*, 7, 265, 1909.
Carrel, A. Technique for Cultivating a Large Quantity of Tissue. *J. Exper. Med.*, 15, 393, 1912.
——— Man, the Unknown. New York and London, Harper & Brothers, 1935.
Clunet, J. Recherches Expérimentales sur les Tumeurs Malignes. Paris, Steinheil, 1910.
Contamin, A. Le cancer expérimental: Revue des travaux récents, recherches personelles. Paris, Masson et Cie, 1910. (Bibliography on transplanted cancer.)
Cornil. Cited by Woglom, p. 49.
Coste, G. Recherches expérimentales sur le sarcome de Jensen. Thèse d'Alger, 1934. Abstract in *Index Analyt. Cancerol.*, 9, 28, 1935.
de Martel, T. A propos de l'évolution du cancer. *Bull. et Mém. Soc. Nat. de Chirurg.*, 60, 1390, 1934.
Durand. Cited by Woglom, p. 43.
Ehrlich, P. Experimentelle Studien an Mäusetumoren. *Ztschr. f. Krebsforsch.*, 5, 59, 1907.

Ehrlich, P., and Apolant, H. Beobachtungen über maligne Mäusetumoren. *Berliner klin. Wchnschr.*, 62, 871, 1905.

Fayet. Cited by Woglom, p. 43.

Fouts, P. J., Corcoran, A. C., and Page, I. H. Observations on the Clinical and Functional Course of Nephrotoxic Nephritis in Dogs. *American J. Med. Sci.*, 201, 313, 1941. (Literature on nephrotoxic sera.)

Greene, H. S. N. Heterologous Transplantation of Mammalian Tumors. II. The Transfer of Human Tumors to Alien Species. *J. Exper. Med.*, 73, 475, 1941.

Haaland, M. Les Tumeurs de la Souris. *Ann. Inst. Pasteur,* 19, 129, 1905.

——— Contributions to the Study of the Development of Sarcoma under Experimental Conditions. Third Scientific Report, Imperial Cancer Research Fund. London, Taylor & Francis, 1908.

Hahn. Cited by Woglom, p. 48.

Hanau, A. Erfolgreiche experimentelle Uebertragung von Carcinom. *Fortschritte der Med.*, 7, 321, 1889.

Harrison, R. B. Observations on the living developing nerve fiber. *Proc. Soc. Exper. Biol. and Med.*, 4, 140, 1907.

Heidenhain, L. Ist Krebs durch Zerfallsprodukte übertragbar? *Ztschr. f. Krebsforsch.*, 36, 360, 1932.

Heiman, J. The Study of Benign Neoplasms of the Rat's Breast. *American J. Cancer,* 22, 497, 1934.

Héricourt, J., and Richet, C. De la Sérotherapie dans le traitement du cancer. *Compt. rend. Acad. Sci.*, 121, 567, 1895.

Hirschfeld, H. Ueber Heil- und Immunisierungsvorgänge an Tumortieren. *Ztschr. f. Krebsforsch.*, 16, 93, 1919.

Jensen, C. O. Experimentelle Untersuchungen über Krebs bei Mäusen. *Centralbl. f. Bakteriol.*, etc., Abt. I., 34, 28, 122, 1903.

Le Noble. Cited by Woglom, p. 43.

Lewin, C. Experimentelle Beiträge zur Morphologie und Biologie bösartiger Geschwülste bei Ratten und Mäusen. *Ztschr. f. Krebsforsch.*, 6, 267, 1908.

Loeb, Leo. On Transplantation of Tumors. *J. Med. Research.*, n.s., 1, 28, 1901.

——— Ueber Sarkomentwicklung bei einem drüsenartigen Mäusetumor. *Berliner klin. Wchnschr.*, 43, 798, 1906.

Lumsden, T. Tumour Immunity. *American J. Cancer,* 15, 563, 1931.

Masugi, M. Über die experimentelle Glomerulonephritis durch das spezifische Antinierenserum. *Beitr. z. path. Anat. u. z. allg. Pathol.*, 92, 429, 1933–34.

Morau, H. Inoculation en série d'une tumeur épithéliale de la souris blanche. *Compt. rend. Soc. Biol.*, 43, 289, 1891.

Murphy, J. B. Transplantability of Tissues to the Embryo of Foreign Species. *J. Exper. Med.*, 17, 482, 1913.

Nagayo, M. On Heteroplastic Transplantation of Mouse Sarcoma. *Gann,* 35, 232, 1941.

Oberling, C., Guérin, M., and Guérin, P. A propos de la transformation sarcomateuse des fibroadénomes mammaires transplantables du rat blanc. *Bull. Assn. Française pour l'Etude du Cancer.* 24, 232, 1935.

Peyrilhe, B. A Dissertation on Cancerous Diseases. London, 1775.

Putnoky, J. Über die heteroplastische Transplantation des Ehrlichschen überimpfbaren Mäusecarcinoms. *Ztschr. f. Krebsforsch.*, 32, 520, 1930.

Roessle, R. Fortschritte der Cytotoxinforschung. *Ergebnisse d. allg. Pathol. u. pathol. Anat.*, 13, 124, 1909.

Roussy, G., Oberling, C., and Guérin, M. La rôle de l'ablation des tumeurs greffées dans la production des métastases. Libro de Oro dedicado al Prof. Dr. Angel H. Roffo. 1910–35. P. 1209.

Russell, B. R. G. Sarcoma Development Occurring During the Propagation of a Haemorrhagic Adeno-carcinoma of the Mamma of the Mouse. *J. Pathol. and Bacteriol.*, 14, 344, 1910.

Saphir, O., and Appel, M. Regression of Primary Brown-Pearce Testicular Carcinoma and Metastases Following Intracutaneous Transplantation with Homologous Tumor. *American J. Cancer,* 38, 55, 1940.
Strong, L. C. Genetic Indications Correlated with the Transplantation of Cancerous Tissue. *J. Heredity,* 15, 355, 1924.
——— Transplantation Studies on Tumors Arising Spontaneously in Heterozygous Individuals. *J. Cancer Research,* 13, 103, 1929.
Voegtlin, C. Biochemistry of Malignant Tissues. *Physiological Reviews,* 17, 92, 1937.
von Wassermann, A., Keysser, F., and Wassermann, M. Beiträge zum Problem: Geschwülste von der Blutbahn aus therapeutisch zu beeinflussen. *Deutsche med. Wchnschr.,* 37, 2389, 1911.
Woglom, W. H. Mice Immunized Subcutaneously are Resistant to the Implantation of Cancer in Internal Organs. *Lancet,* 2, 92, 1911.
——— The Study of Experimental Cancer: A Review. New York, Columbia University Press, 1913.
——— Immunity to Transplantable Tumours. *Cancer Review,* 4, 129, 1929. (Bibliography.)

CARCINOGENIC RAYS

Andervont, H. B., and Shimkin, M. B. Tumors in Mice Injected with Colloidal Thorium Dioxide. *J. National Cancer Inst.,* 1, 349, 1940.
Bang, F. Le cancer des cicatrices. Etude clinique et expérimentale. *Bull. Assoc. Française pour l'Etude du Cancer,* 14, 203, 1925.
Beard, H. H., Boggess, T. S., and von Haam, E. Experimental Production of Malignant Tumors in the Albino Rat by Means of Ultraviolet Rays. *American J. Cancer,* 27, 257, 1936.
Bloch, B. Die experimentelle Erzeugung von Röntgencarcinomen beim Kaninchen, nebst allgemeinen Bemerkungen über die Genese der experimentelle Carcinome. *Schweizerische med. Wchnschr.,* 54, 857, 1924.
Blum, H. F. Sunlight and Cancer of the Skin. *J. National Cancer Inst.,* 1, 397, 1940–41. (Bibliography.)
Clunet, J. Recherches expérimentales sur les tumeurs malignes. Paris, Steinheil, 1910.
Cornil, L., Paillas, J. E., and Bonneau, H. Le cancer des brûlures. *Bull. Assn. française pour l'Etude du Cancer,* 28, 359, 1939. (Bibliography.)
Daels, F. Experimentelle bösartige Geschwülste. *Arch. klin. Chirurgie,* 177, 144, 1933.
——— and Biltris, R. Contribution à l'étude de la provocation de tumeurs malignes expérimentales au moyen de substances radio-actives. *Bull. Assoc. française pour l'Etude du Cancer,* 20, 32, 1931.
Feygin, Sophie. Du cancer radiologique. Thèse de Paris, 1914.
Findlay, G. M. Ultra-Violet Light and Skin Cancer. *Lancet,* 2, 1070, 1928.
——— Cutaneous Papillomata in the Rat Following Exposure to Ultra-Violet Light. *Lancet,* 1, 1229, 1930.
Foulds, L. The Production of Transplantable Carcinoma and Sarcoma in Guinea Pigs by Injections of Thorotrast. *American J. Cancer,* 35, 363, 1939.
Frieben. Cancroid des rechten Handrückens. *Deutsche med. Wchnschr.,* 28, Vereins-Beilage 335, 1902.
Grady, H. G., Blum, H. F., and Kirby-Smith, J. S. Histologic Changes in the Skin of Mice Following Radiation from Mercury Arc. *American J. Pathol.,* 17, 446, 1941.
Hartwell, J. L. Survey of Compounds Which Have Been Tested for Carcinogenic Activity. Federal Security Agency: United States Public Health Service, 1941. (Bibliography.)
Hellner, H. Ueber Strahlengeschwülste. Experimentell erzeugtes Knochensarkom. *Münchener med. Wchnschr.,* 84, 980, 1937.
Henshaw, P. S. Further Studies on Action of Roentgen Rays on Gametes of *Arbacia*

punctulata; Production of Multipolar Cleavage in Eggs by Exposure of Gametes to Roentgen Rays. *American J. Roentgenol. and Radium Therapy*, 43, 923, 1940.

Herlitz, C. W., Jundell, J., and Wahlgren, F. Durch Ultraviolettbestrahlung erzeugte maligne Neubildungen bei weissen Mäusen. *Acta paediatr.*, 10, 321, 1931.

Huldschinsky, K. Augensarkome bei Ratten hervorgerufen durch abnorm lange Ultravioletteinwirkung. *Deutsche med. Wchnschr.*, 59, 530, 1933.

Jonkhoff, A. R. Röntgencarcinom bei Mäusen. *Ztschr. f. Krebsforsch.*, 26, 32, 1927.

Lacassagne, A., and Vinzent, R. Sarcomes provoqués chez des Lapins par l'irradiation d'abcès à *Streptobacillus caviae. Compt. rend. Soc. Biol.*, 100, 249, 1929.

Lüdin, M. Knochensarkom nach experimenteller Röntgenbestrahlung. *Acta Radiologica*, 15, 553, 1934.

Martland, H. S. The Occurrence of Malignancy in Radioactive Persons. *American J. Cancer*, 15, 2435, 1931.

Muller, H. J. The Effects of Roentgen Rays upon the Hereditary Material. The Science of Radiology. O. Glasser. Baltimore, Charles C. Thomas, 1933.

Oberling, C., and Guérin, M. Action du thorotrast sur le sarcome de Jensen du rat blanc. *Bull. Assn. Française pour l'Etude du Cancer*, 22, 469, 1933.

Putschar, W., and Holtz, F. Erzeugung von Hautkrebsen bei Ratten durch langdauernde Ultraviolettbestrahlung. *Ztschr. f. Krebsforsch.*, 33, 219, 1930.

Roffo, A. H. Krebs und Sarkom durch Ultraviolett- und Sonnenbestrahlen. *Ztschr. f. Krebsforsch.*, 41, 448, 1935.

Roussy, G., Oberling, C., and Guérin, M. Action cancerigène du dioxyde de thorium chez le rat blanc. *Bull. Acad. Méd.*, Paris, 112, 809, 1934.

Rusch, H. P., and Baumann, C. A. Tumor Production in Mice with Ultraviolet Irradiation. *American J. Cancer*, 35, 55, 1939.

Sabin, Florence R., Doan, C. A., and Forkner, C. E. The Production of Osteogenic Sarcomata and the Effects on Lymph Nodes and Bone Marrow of Intravenous Injections of Radium Chloride and Mesothorium in Rabbits. *J. Exper. Med.*, 56, 267, 1932.

Schürch, O., and Uehlinger, E. Über experimentelle Erzeugung von Knochensarkomen mit Radium und Mesothorium. *Bull. schweiz. Vereinigung Krebsbekämpfung*, 3, 271, 1936. Abstract in *Ztschr. f. Krebsforsch.*, 48, Ref. 18, 1939.

Selbie, F. R. Tumours in Rats and Mice Following Injection of Thorotrast. *British J. Exper. Pathol.*, 19, 100, 1938.

Timoféeff-Ressovsky, N. W. Experimentelle Mutationsforschung in der Vererbungslehre: Beeinflussung der Erbanlagen durch Strahlung und andere Faktoren. Wissenschaftl. Forschungsberichte. R. E. Liesegang, editor. Naturwissenschaftl. Reihe, 42. Leipzig and Dresden, Steinkopf, 1937.

Uehlinger, E., and Schürch, O. Über experimentelle Erzeugung von Sarkomen mit Radium und Mesothorium. *Deutsche Ztschr. f. Chirurgie*, 251, 12, 1938.

PARASITES AS A CAUSE OF CANCER

Askanazy, M. Distomum felineum beim Menschen in Ostpreussen. *Verhandl. d. deutschen pathol. Gesellsch.*, 3, 72, 1900.

Bonne, C. Cancer of the stomach of wild rat and infection with nematode worm, Hepaticola gastrica Baylis, 1925. *J. Tropical Med.*, 29, 288, 1926.

——— and Sandground, J. H. On the Production of Gastric Tumors, Bordering on Malignancy, in Javanese Monkeys through the Agency of *Nochtia nochti*, a Parasitic Nematode. *American J. Cancer*, 37, 173, 1939.

Borrel, A. Observations étiologiques. *Ztschr. f. Krebsforsch.*, 5, 106, 1907.

——— Le problème étiologique du Cancer. *Ztschr. f. Krebsforsch.*, 7, 265, 1909.

——— Acariens et cancers. *Ann. Inst. Pasteur*, 23, 97, 1909.

——— Cited by Fibiger. *Ztschr. f. Krebsforsch.*, 13, 217, 1913.

Borrel, A. Die Ätiologie der bösartigen Geschwülste. *Ztschr. f. Krebsforsch.*, 32, 646, 1930.
Brumpt, E. Précis de Parasitologie. 5th ed. Paris, Masson et Cie., 1936.
Brunschwig, A., and Rasmussen, R. A. The Relation of Diet to Benign Neoplasia (Ulcero-Papillomas) of the Rat's Stomach. *Cancer Research*, 1, 371, 1941.
Bullock, F. D., and Curtis, M. R. A Study of the Reactions of the Tissues of the Rat's Liver to the Larvae of *Taenia Crassicollis* and the Histogenesis of Cysticercus Sarcoma. *J. Cancer Research*, 8, 446, 1924.
Cramer, W. Twenty-Sixth Annual Report, Imperial Cancer Research Fund. 1927–1928. P. 8.
——— Papillomatosis in the Forestomach of the Rat and its Bearing on the Work of Fibiger. *American J. Cancer*, 31, 537, 1937.
Curtis, M. R., Dunning, W. F., and Bullock, F. D. Genetic Factors in Relation to the Etiology of Malignant Tumors. *American J. Cancer*, 17, 894, 1933.
——— ——— ——— Further Evidence in Support of the Somatic Mutation Hypothesis of the Origin of Malignancy. *American J. Cancer*, 21, 86, 1934.
——— ——— ——— Duration and Extent of Irritation versus Genetic Constitution in the Etiology of Malignant Tumors. *J. Cancer Research*, 21, 554, 1934.
Dunning, W. F., and Curtis, M. R. Malignancy Induced by *Cysticercus Fasciolaris*: Its Independence of the Age of the Host when Infested. *American J. Cancer*, 37, 312, 1939.
Falko. Cited by Brumpt.
Fibiger, J. Untersuchungen über eine Nematode und deren Fähigkeit, papillomatöse und carcinomatöse Geschwulstbildungen im Magen der Ratte hervorzurufen. *Ztschr. f. Krebsforsch.*, 13, 217, 1913.
——— Untersuchungen über das Spiropterakarzinom der Ratte und der Maus. *Ztschr. f. Krebsforsch.*, 17, 1, 1920.
Fielding. Cited by Brumpt.
Fridericia, L. S., Gudjonsson, S., Vimtrup, B., Clemmesen, S., and Clemmesen, J. Stomach Lesions in Rats Kept on Diets Deficient in Vitamin A. *American J. Cancer*, 39, 61, 1940.
Fujimaki, Y. Formation of Gastric Carcinoma in Albino Rats Fed on Deficient Diets. *J. Cancer Research*, 10, 469, 1926.
——— Arimoto, K., Kimura, T., Ohba, K., and Matsuda, G. On the Morphological Changes of the Forestomach of Albino Rats due to Feeding of Specific Diets. V. Relationship between the Grade of Morphological Changes in the Forestomach and the Kinds of Fats. *Trans. Japanese Pathol. Soc.*, 21, 708, 1931.
Galeb, O. Observations et expériences sur les migrations du Filaria rytipleuritis. *Compt. rend. Acad. Sci.*, 87, 75, 1878.
McCoy, G. W. A Preliminary Report on Tumors Found in Wild Rats. *J. Med. Research*, n.s., 16, 285, 1909.
Nishimura. Cited by Brumpt.
Pappenheimer, A. M., and Larrimore, L. D. The Occurrence of Gastric Lesions in Rats: Their Relation to Dietary Deficiency and Hair Ingestion. *J. Exper. Med.*, 40, 719, 1924.
Passey, R. D., Leese, A., and Knox, J. C. Spiroptera Cancer and Diet Deficiency. *J. Pathol. and Bacteriol.*, 40, 198, 1935.
Seurat. Cited by Brumpt.
Strong, R. P. The Rôle Played by Helminths in the Production of Tumors in Man and Animals. *International Clinics*, 4, 68, 1931.
Sugiura, K. The Relation of Diet to the Development of Gastric Lesions in the Rat. *Cancer Research*, 2, 770, 1942. (Bibliography.)
Tubangui. Cited by Brumpt.
Virchow, R. Medicinische Erinnerungen von einer Reise nach Aegypten. *Virch. Arch.*, 113, 361, 1888.
Yokogawa. Cited by Brumpt.

HEREDITARY FACTORS IN CANCER

AHLBOM, H. E. Simple Achlorhydric Anaemia, Plummer-Vinson Syndrome, and Carcinoma of the Mouth, Pharynx, and Oesophagus in Women. *British Med. J.*, 2, 331, 1936.

CLOUDMAN, A. M., and LITTLE, C. C. The Genetics of Tumour Formation in Mice, in Relation to the Gene T for Brachyury. *J. Genetics*, 32, 487, 1936.

CRAMER, W. On the Aetiology of Cancer of the Mamma in the Mouse and in Man. *American J. Cancer*, 30, 318, 1937.

DOBROVOLSKAIA-ZAVADSKAIA, N. Heredity of Cancer. *American J. Cancer*, 18, 357, 1933. (Bibliography.)

GORER, P. A. The Genetics of Cancer in the Mouse. *Lancet*, 2, 461, 1937.

GREENE, H. S. N. Familial Mammary Tumors in the Rabbit. *J. Exper. Med.*, 70, 147, 159, 167, 1939.

KORTEWEG, R. Chromosomale invloeden op den groei en extrachromosomale invloeden op het ontstaan van kanker bij de muis. *Nederl. tijdschr. v. geneesk.*, 79, 1482, 1935.

KREYBERG, L. On the Susceptibility to Cancer Development in the Skin and in the Mammary Gland in Two Lines of Inbred Mice. *American J. Cancer*, 24, 554, 1935.

LATHROP, A. E. C., and LOEB, LEO. The incidence of cancer in various strains of mice. *Proc. Soc. Exper. Biol. and Med.*, 11, 34, 1913–14.

LITTLE, C. C. The Constitutional Factor in the Incidence of Mammary Tumors. *American J. Cancer*, 27, 551, 1936.

——— MURRAY, W. S., and CLOUDMAN, A. M. The Genetics of Non-Epithelial Tumor Formation in Mice. *American J. Cancer*, 36, 431, 1939.

LYNCH, CLARA J. Studies on the Relation between Tumor Susceptibility and Heredity. I. *J. Exper. Med.*, 39, 481, 1924.

——— Studies on the Relation between Tumor Susceptibility and Heredity. VI. Lung Tumors in Mice with Respect to the Phenomenon of Maternal Influence. *American J. Cancer*, 31, 77, 1937.

MARSH, M. C. Spontaneous Mammary Cancer in Mice. *J. Cancer Research*, 13, 313, 1929.

MACDOWELL, E. C., and RICHTER, M. N. Mouse Leukemia. IX. The Rôle of Heredity in Spontaneous Cases. *Arch. Pathol.*, 20, 709, 1935.

MCFARLAND, J., and MEADE, T. S. The Genetic Origin of Tumors Supported by their Simultaneous and Symmetrical Occurrence in Homologous Twins. *American J. Med. Sci.*, n.s., 184, 66, 1932. (Bibliography.)

MURRAY, J. A. Cancerous Ancestry and the Incidence of Cancer in Mice. Fourth Scientific Report, Imperial Cancer Research Fund. London, Taylor & Francis, 1911.

MURRAY, W. S. Factors Influencing the Incidence of Mammary Gland Tumors in an Inbred Strain of Mice. *J. Cancer Research*, 14, 602, 1930.

——— and LITTLE, C. C. Chromosomal and Extrachromosomal Influence in Relation to the Incidence of Mammary Tumors in Mice. *American J. Cancer*, 37, 536, 1939.

PAULSEN, J. Konstitution und Krebs. *Ztschr. f. Krebsforsch.*, 21, 119, 1924.

PEYRON, A., and KOBOZIEFF, N. Les tumeurs chez les jumeaux. *Bull. Assn. française pour l'Etude du Cancer*, 26, 93, 1937.

——— ——— and ZIMMER, L. Sur l'hérédité de la neurofibromatose. *Bull. Assn. Française pour l'Etude du Cancer*, 26, 168, 1937.

PLUMMER. Cited by Vinson.

SLYE, MAUD. The Incidence and Inheritability of Spontaneous Tumors in Mice. (Second Report.) *J. Med. Research*, n.s., 25, 281, 1914.

——— The Incidence and Inheritability of Spontaneous Cancer in Mice. (Third Report.) *J. Med. Research*, n.s., 27, 159, 1915.

——— The Inheritability of Spontaneous Tumors of Specific Organs and of Specific Types in Mice. (Fifth Report.) *J. Cancer Research*, 1, 479, 1916.

Slye, Maud. The Inheritability of Spontaneous Tumors of the Liver in Mice. (Seventh Report.) *J. Cancer Research*, 1, 503, 1916.

——— The Influence of Heredity in Determining Tumor Metastases. (Sixteenth Report.) *J. Cancer Research*, 6, 139, 1921.

——— Biological Evidence for the Inheritability of Cancer in Man. (Eighteenth Report.) *J. Cancer Research*, 7, 107, 1922.

——— L'hérédité dans le cancer. *Bull. Assn. Française pour l'Etude du Cancer*, 26, 138, 1937.

Snell, G. D. (Editor). Mouse Genetic News. Bar Harbor, Roscoe B. Jackson Memorial Laboratory, 1941. No. 1, November. (Extensive list of inbred strains of mice.)

Strong, L. C. General Considerations on the Genetic Study of Cancer. *J. Cancer Research*, 10, 219, 1926.

——— Transplantation Studies on Tumors Arising Spontaneously in Heterozygous Individuals. I. Experimental Evidence for the Theory that the Tumor Cell has Deviated from a Definitive Somatic Cell by a Process Analogous to Genetic Mutation. *J. Cancer Research*, 13, 103, 1929.

Tyzzer, E. E. A Study of Heredity in Relation to the Development of Tumors in Mice. *J. Med. Research*, n.s., 12, 199, 1907–08.

Versluys, J. J. Zwillingspathologischer Beitrag zur Ätiologie der Tumoren. *Ztschr. f. Krebsforsch.*, 41, 239, 1935.

Vinson, P. P. Hysterical Dysphagia. *Minnesota Med.*, 5, 107, 1922.

Waaler, G. H. M. Über die Erblichkeit des Krebses. Oslo, Dybwad, 1931.

Warthin, A. S. Heredity with Reference to Carcinoma. *Arch. Internal Med.*, 12, 546, 1913.

——— The Further Study of a Cancer Family. *J. Cancer Research*, 9, 279, 1925.

——— The Nature of Cancer Susceptibility in Human Families. *J. Cancer Research*, 12, 249, 1928.

Wassink, W. F. Cancer et hérédité. *Genetica*, 17, 103, 1935.

——— International Cancer Congress, Brussels, 1936. Communications, p. 171.

THE TAR TUMOR

Bayon, H. Epithelial Proliferation Induced by the Injection of Gasworks Tar. *Lancet*, 2, 1579, 1912.

Beck, S. Experimentelle Erzeugung einer Disposition zum Teerkrebs an Tieren. *Ztschr. f. Krebsforsch.*, 24, 278, 1927.

Cazin, M. Des origines et des modes de transmission du cancer. Paris, 1894.

Fischer-Wasels, B. Die physiologischen Grundlagen der allgemeinen Geschwulstdisposition. *Virch. Arch.*, 275, 723, 1929.

Flory, C. M. The Production of Tumors by Tobacco Tars. *Cancer Research*, 1, 262, 1941.

Haga, I. Experimentelle Untersuchungen über die Erzeugung atypischer Epithel- und Schleimhautwucherungen. *Ztschr. f. Krebsforsch.* 12, 525, 1913. (Bibliography.)

Hanau, A. Erfolgreiche experimentelle Uebertragung von Carcinom. *Fortschritte der Med.*, 7, 321, 1889.

Hueper, W. C. Occupational Tumors and Allied Diseases. Springfield and Baltimore, Thomas, 1942. (Bibliography.)

Maisin, J. Le Cancer du goudron est-il simplement un cancer d'irritation locale? *Compt. rend. Congrès du Cancer*, 26, Strasbourg, 1923.

——— and Masse, G. Le cancer du goudron est-il simplement un cancer d'irritation locale? *Compt. rend. Soc. Biol.*, 93, 449, 1925.

Murphy, J. B., and Sturm, E. Primary Lung Tumors in Mice Following the Cutaneous Application of Coal Tar. *J. Exper. Med.*, 42, 693, 1925.

Oberling, C., and Raileanu, C. Proliférations papillomateuses de l'orielle du lapin provoquées par injections intratrachéales d'huile de vaseline goudronnée. *Bull. Assn. française pour l'Etude du Cancer*, 20, 90, 1931.

POTT, PERCIVALL. Chirurgical Observations Relative to the Cataract, the Polypus of the Nose, the Cancer of the Scrotum, the Different Kinds of Ruptures, and the Mortification of the Toes and Feet. London, Carnegy, 1775.

REDING, R., and SLOSSE, A. Des caractères généraux de l'état cancéreux et précancéreux. *Bull. Assn. Française pour l'Etude du Cancer*, 18, 122, 1929.

ROFFO, A. H. Durch Tabak beim Kaninchen entwickeltes Carcinom. *Ztschr. f. Krebsforsch.*, 33, 321, 1931.

SCHABAD, L. M. Über operative Entfernung des experimentellen Teerkrebses und dessen Vorstufen und die Fernresultate derselben. *Ztschr. f. Krebsforsch.*, 31, 621, 1930.

SCHÜRCH, O., and WINTERSTEIN, A. Experimentelle Untersuchungen zur Frage Tabak und Krebs. *Ztschr. f. Krebsforsch.*, 42, 76, 1935.

SEELIG, M. G., and COOPER, Z. K. A Review of the Recent Literature of Tar Cancer (1927–1931 inclusive). *American J. Cancer*, 17, 589, 1933. (Bibliography.)

TSUTSUI, H. Ueber das künstlich erzeugte Cancroid bei der Maus. *Gann*, 12, 17, 1918.

WOGLOM, W. H. Experimental Tar Cancer. *Arch. Pathol.*, 2, 533, 709, 1926. (Bibliography.)

YAMAGIWA, K., and ICHIKAWA, K. Experimental Study of the Pathogenesis of Carcinoma. *J. Cancer Research*, 3, 1, 1918.

THE CARCINOGENIC HYDROCARBONS

ALLEN, E., and GARDNER, W. U. Cancer of the Cervix of the Uterus in Hybrid Mice Following the Long-Continued Administration of Estrogen. *Cancer Research*, 1, 359, 1941.

ANDERVONT, H. B. Pulmonary Tumors in Mice. IV. Lung Tumors Induced by Subcutaneous Injection of 1:2:5:6-Dibenzanthracene in Different Media and by its Direct Contact with Lung Tissues. *Public Health Rep.*, 52, 1584, 1937.

ANDO, T. Einfluss der Futtermittel auf die experimentelle Leberkarzinomentstehung. (I. Mitteilung.) Experimentelle Leberkarzinomentstehung mit Getreide (Zeitdauer d. Fütterung: 280 Tage). *Gann*, 34, 371, 1940.

ANISSIMOVA, V. Experimental Zinc Teratomas of the Testis and their Transplantation. Preliminary Communication. *American J. Cancer*, 36, 229, 1939.

BERENBLUM, I. The Cocarcinogenic Action of Croton Resin. *Cancer Research*, 1, 44, 1941.

BLOCH, B., and DREIFUSS, W. Ueber die experimentelle Erzeugung von Carcinom mit Lymphdrüsen- und Lungenmetastasen. *Schweizerische med. Wchnschr.*, 51, 1033, 1921.

BONSER, GEORGIANA M. Malignant Tumours of the Interstitial Cells of the Testis in Strong A Mice Treated with Triphenylethylene. *J. Pathol. and Bacteriol.*, 54, 149, 1942.

——— Epithelial Tumours of the Bladder in Dogs Induced by Pure β-Naphthylamine. *J. Pathol. and Bacteriol.*, 55, 1, 1943.

——— and ROBSON, J. M. The Effects of Prolonged Oestrogen Administration upon Male Mice of Various Strains: Development of Testicular Tumours in the Strong A Strain. *J. Pathol. and Bacteriol.*, 51, 9, 1940.

BROWNING, C. H., GULBRANSEN, R., and NIVEN, J. S. F. Sarcoma Production in Mice by Single Subcutaneous Injection of a Benzoylamino Quinoline Styryl Compound. *J. Pathol. and Bacteriol.*, 42, 155, 1936.

BURROWS, H. Carcinoma Mammae Occurring in a Male Mouse under Continued Treatment with Oestrin. *American J. Cancer*, 24, 613, 1935.

CHAMPY, C., and LAVEDAN, J. P. Seminomes par régénérations testiculaires chez les oiseaux. *Bull. Assn. Française pour l'Etude du Cancer*, 28, 503, 1939.

COOK, J. W., DODDS, E. C., and LAWSON, W. Further Observations on Oestrogenic

Activity of Synthetic Polycyclic Compounds. *Proc. Roy. Soc.*, London, Series B, 121, 133, 1936.

Cook, J. W., Haslewood, G. A. D., Hewett, C. L., Hieger, I., Kennaway, E. L., and Mayneord, W. V. Chemical Compounds as Carcinogenic Agents. *American J. Cancer*, 29, 219, 1937. (Bibliography.)

——— Hewett, C. L., and Hieger, I. The Isolation of a Cancer-Producing Hydrocarbon from Coal Tar. Parts I, II, and III. Part I. Concentration of the Active Substance. By I. Hieger. *J. Chemical Soc.*, p. 395, 1933.

——— and Kennaway, E L. Chemical Compounds as Carcinogenic Agents. First Supplementary Report: Literature of 1937. *American J. Cancer*, 33, 50, 1938. (Bibliography.)

——— ——— Chemical Compounds as Carcinogenic Agents. Second Supplementary Report: Literature of 1938 and 1939. *American J. Cancer*, 39, 381, 521, 1940. (Bibliography.)

Cramer, W., and Horning, E. S. Experimental Production by Oestrin of Pituitary Tumours with Hypopituitarism and of Mammary Cancer. *Lancet*, 1, 247, 1936.

Deelman, H. T. Ueber experimentelle maligne Geschwülste durch Teereinwirkung bei Mäusen. *Ztschr. f. Krebsforsch.*, 18, 261, 1922.

des Ligneris, M. J. A. The Production of Benign and Malignant Skin Tumours in Mice Painted with Bantu Liver Extracts. *American J. Cancer*, 39, 489, 1940.

Engelbreth-Holm, J., and Lefèvre, H. Acceleration of the Development of Leukemias and Mammary Carcinomas in Mice by 9, 10-Dimethyl-1, 2-Benzanthracene. *Cancer Research*, 1, 102, 1941.

Falin, L. I., and Gromzewa, K. E. Experimental Teratoma Testis in Fowl Produced by Injections of Zinc Sulphate Solution. Preliminary Communication. *American J. Cancer*, 36, 233, 1939.

Fieser, L. F. Carcinogenic Activity, Structure, and Chemical Reactivity of Polynuclear Aromatic Hydrocarbons. *American J. Cancer*, 34, 37, 1938. (Bibliography.)

Fischer, B. Ueber experimentelle Erzeugung von Epithelwucherung und Epithelmetaplasie. *Verhandl. d. Deutschen Pathol. Gesellsch.*, 10, 20, 1906.

Flory, C. M. The Production of Tumors by Tobacco Tars. *Cancer Research*, 1, 262, 1941.

Furth, J., and Furth, O. B. Monocytic Leukemia and Other Neoplastic Diseases Occurring in Mice Following Intrasplenic Injection of 1:2-Benzpyrene. *American J. Cancer*, 34, 169, 1938.

Gardner, W. U. Estrogens in Carcinogenesis. *Arch. Pathol.*, 27, 138, 1939. (Bibliography.)

——— Smith, G. M., Allen, E., and Strong, L. C. Cancer of the Mammary Glands in Male Mice Receiving Estrogenic Hormone. *Arch. Pathol.*, 21, 265, 1936.

Geschickter, C. F. Mammary Carcinoma in Rat with Metastasis Induced by Estrogen. *Science*, 89, 35, 1939.

Hieger, I. The Spectra of Cancer-Producing Tars and Oils and of Related Substances. *Biochemical J.*, 24, 505, 1930.

——— The Examination of Human Tissue for Carcinogenic Factors. *American J. Cancer*, 39, 496, 1940.

——— See also Cook, Hewett, and Hieger.

Hueper, W. C., Wiley, F. H., and Wolfe, H. D. Experimental Production of Bladder Tumors in Dogs by Administration of Betanaphthylamine. *J. Indust. Hyg. and Toxicol.*, 20, 46, 1938.

Kennaway, E. L. The Formation of a Cancer-Producing Substance from Isoprene (2-methylbutadiene). *J. Pathol. and Bacteriol.*, 27, 233, 1924.

——— and Hieger, I. Carcinogenic Substances and their Fluorescence Spectra. *British Med. J.*, 1, 1044, 1930.

Kinosita, R. Special Report. Studies on the Carcinogenic Chemical Substances. *Trans. Japanese Pathol. Soc.*, 27, 665, 1937.

KINOSITA, R. Studies on Cancerogenic Chemical Substances. *J. Japan Soc. Diseases Digestive Organs,* 37, 513, 1938.
——— On the substances to affect the experimental cancerogenesis. (In Japanese.) Cited by Sugiura and Benedict.
——— Studies on the Cancerogenic Azo and Related Compounds. *Yale J. Biol. and Med.,* 12, 287, 1940.
KLEINENBERG, H. E., NEUFACH, S. A., and SCHABAD, L. M. Further Study of Blastomogenic Substances in the Human Body. *Cancer Research,* 1, 853, 1941.
LACASSAGNE, A. Apparition de cancers de la mamelle chez la souris mâle soumise à des injections de folliculine. *Compt. rend. Acad. Sci.,* Paris, 195, 630, 1932.
——— Sarcomes fusocellulaires apparus chez des souris longuement traitées par des hormones oestrogènes. *Compt. rend. Soc. Biol.,* 126, 190, 1937.
——— Relationship of Hormones and Mammary Adenocarcinoma in the Mouse. *American J. Cancer,* 37, 414, 1939.
LOEB, LEO. Further Investigations on the Origin of Tumors in Mice. VI. Internal Secretion as a Factor in the Origin of Tumors. *J. Med. Research,* 40, 477, 1919.
——— Estrogenic Hormones and Carcinogenesis. *J. American Med. Assn.,* 104, 1597, 1935. (Bibliography.)
LORENZ, E., and STEWART, H. L. Intestinal Carcinoma and Other Lesions in Mice Following Oral Administration of 1,2,5,6-Dibenzanthracene and 20-Methylcholanthrene. *J. National Cancer Inst.,* 1, 17, 1940–41.
——— ——— Squamous Cell Carcinoma and Other Lesions of the Forestomach in Mice, Following Oral Administration of 20-Methylcholanthrene and 1,2,5,6-Dibenzanthracene. *J. National Cancer Inst.,* 1, 273, 1940–41.
MAISIN, J. Pouvoir cancérigène des sous-produits du goudron. *Bull. Assn. Française pour l'Etude du Cancer,* 12, 488, 1923.
MAYNEORD, W. V. Cited by Hieger. *American J. Cancer,* 29, 705, 1937.
McCOY, G. W. A Preliminary Report on Tumors Found in Wild Rats. *J. Med. Research,* n.s., 16, 285, 1909.
MICHALOWSKY, I. Das 10. experimentelle Zink-Teratom. II. Mitteilung. *Virch. Arch.,* 274, 319, 1929.
MILLER, J. A., MINER, D. L., RUSCH, H. P., and BAUMANN, C. A. Diet and Hepatic Tumor Formation. *Cancer Research,* 1, 699, 1941.
MURPHY, J. B., and STURM, E. Primary Lung Tumors in Mice Following the Cutaneous Application of Coal Tar. *J. Exper. Med.,* 42, 693, 1925.
NAKAHARA, W., FUJIWARA, T., and MORI, K. Inhibiting Effect of Yeast Feeding on the Experimental Production of Liver Cancer. *Gann,* 33, 57, 1939.
NONAKA, T. The Occurrence of Subcutaneous Sarcomas in the Rat after Repeated Injections of Glucose Solution. *Gann,* 32, 234, 1938.
OBERLING, C., GUÉRIN, M., and GUÉRIN, P. Particularités évolutives des tumeurs produites avec de fortes doses de benzopyrène. *Bull. Assn. Française pour l'Etude du Cancer,* 28, 198, 1939.
——— SANNIÉ, C., GUÉRIN, M., and GUÉRIN, P. Recherches sur l'action cancérigène du 1, 2-benzopyrène. *Bull. Assn. Française pour l'Etude du Cancer,* 25, 156, 1936.
——— ——— ——— ——— A propos de l'action cancérigène du benzopyrène. Ve Conference, Leeuwenhoek Vereeniging, Paris, 4, 57, 1937.
OKADA, D. Über den Einfluss der Brotfütterung auf die Leberkarzinomentstehung durch Dimethylaminoazobenzol. *Osaka Igaku Zasshi,* 39, 485, 1940. Cited by Sugiura and Benedict.
OVERHOLSER, M. D., and ALLEN, E. Atypical Growth Induced in Cervical Epithelium of the Monkey by Prolonged Injections of Ovarian Hormone Combined with Chronic Trauma. *Surgery, Gynecol., and Obstet.,* 60, 129, 1935.
PERLMANN, S., and STAEHLER, W. Über künstlich erzeugte Geschwülste der Blase. *Klin. Wchnschr.,* 11, 1955, 1932.
PIERSON, HANNAH. Weitere Follikulinversuche. Perforierende Plattenepithelwucher-

ungen im Uterus des Kaninchens mit Knorpel- und Knochenbefunden. *Ztschr. f. Krebsforsch.* 47, 1, 1937.

REHN, L. Blasengeschwülste bei Fuchsin-Arbeitern. *Arch. f. klin. Chirurgie,* 50, 588, 1895.

ROFFO, A. H. Rôle of Ultra-Violet Rays in the Development of Cancer Provoked by the Sun. *Lancet,* 1, 472, 1936.

ROSS, H. C. Occupational Cancer. *J. Cancer Research,* 3, 321, 1918.

——— and CROPPER, J. W. Gasworks Pitch Industries and Cancer. London, 1913.

ROUS, P., and KIDD, J. G. Conditional Neoplasms and Subthreshold Neoplastic States: A Study of the Tar Tumors of Rabbits. *J. Exper. Med.,* 73, 365, 1941.

SANNIÉ, C., TRUHAUT, R., and GUÉRIN, P. Production de sarcomes chez la souris par injections d'un extrait obtenu à partir de foies de malades cancéreux. *Bull. Assn. Française pour l'Etude du Cancer,* 29, 106, 1940–41.

SASAKI, T., and YOSHIDA, T. Experimentelle Erzeugung des Leberkarzinoms durch Fütterung mit o-Amidoazotoluol. *Virch. Arch.,* 295, 175, 1935.

SCHABAD, L. M. Nouvelles données relatives à l'obtention expérimentale des tumeurs par un extrait benzénique du foie d'un cancéreux. A propos des substances blastogènes endogènes. *Compt. rend. Soc. Biol.,* 126, 1180, 1937.

——— Quelques données expérimentales sur les tumeurs du poumon. *Arch. biol. Nauk,* 51, 16, 1938. Abstract in *Ztschr. f. Krebsforsch.,* 49, Ref. 103, 1940.

SCHÄR, W. Experimentelle Erzeugung von Blasentumoren. (Die Wirkung langdauernder Inhalation von aromatischen Amidoverbindungen.) *Deutsche Ztschr. f. Chirurgie,* 226, 81, 1930.

SELYE, H., THOMSON, D. L., and COLLIP, J. B. Metaplasia of Uterine Epithelium Produced by Chronic Oestrin Administration. *Nature,* London, 135, 65, 1935.

SHEAR, M. J. Studies in Carcinogenesis. I. The Production of Tumors in Mice with Hydrocarbons. *American J. Cancer,* 26, 322, 1936.

——— Studies in Carcinogenesis. IV. Development of Liver Tumors in Pure Strain Mice Following the Injection of 2-Amino-5-Azotoluene. *American J. Cancer,* 29, 269, 1937.

SOBOTKA, H., and BLOCH, EDITH. Urine Extractives in Cancer. *American J. Cancer,* 35, 50, 1939.

STEINER, P. E. The Induction of Tumors with Extracts from Human Livers and Human Cancers. *Cancer Research,* 2, 425, 1942. (Bibliography.)

SUGIURA, K., and RHOADS, C. P. Experimental Liver Cancer in Rats and Its Inhibition by Rice-Bran Extract, Yeast, and Yeast Extract. *Cancer Research,* 1, 3, 1941.

SUNTZEFF, V., BABCOCK, R. S., and LOEB, LEO. The Development of Sarcoma in Mice Following Long-Continued Injections of a Buffered Solution of Hydrochloric Acid. *American J. Cancer,* 39, 56, 1940.

TAKIZAWA, N. Über die Erzeugung des Sarkoms der Maus und Ratte durch wiederholte subkutane Injectionen der konzentrierten Zuckerlösungen. *Gann,* 32, 236, 1938.

THE CARCINOGENIC VIRUSES

ALLOWAY, J. L. The Transfer in Vitro of R Pneumococci into S Forms of Different Specific Types by the Use of Filtered Pneumococcus Extracts. *J. Exper. Med.,* 55, 91, 1932.

——— Further Observations on the Use of Pneumococcus Extracts in Effecting Transformation of Type in Vitro. *J. Exper. Med.,* 57, 265, 1933.

AMIES, C. R. The Particulate Nature of Avian Sarcoma Agents. *J. Pathol. and Bacteriol.,* 44, 141, 1937.

——— and CARR, J. G. Experiments on the des Ligneris Fowl Sarcoma. With a Note by W. J. Purdy. *American J. Cancer,* 35, 72, 1939.

ANDREWES, C. H. Viruses in Relation to the Aetiology of Tumours. *Lancet,* 2, 63, 117, 1934.

ANDREWES, C. H., and SHOPE, R. E. Changes in Rabbit Fibroma Virus Suggesting Mutation. III. Interpretation of Findings. *J. Exper. Med.*, 63, 179, 1936.

BASSET, J., MACHEBOEF, M., and WOLLMAN, E. Etudes biologiques effectuées grace aux ultrapressions: recherches sur les microbes pathogènes et leurs toxines, sur les virus invisibles, les bactériophages et les tumeurs malignes. *Ann. Inst. Pasteur*, 58, 58, 1937.

BAWDEN, F. C. Plant Viruses and Virus Diseases. Leiden (Chronica Botanica), 1939.

——— and PIRIE, N. W. Liquid Crystalline Preparations of Potato Virus "X." *British J. Exper. Pathol.*, 19, 66, 1938.

——— ——— Crystalline Preparations of Tomato Bushy Stunt Virus. *British J. Exper. Pathol.*, 19, 251, 1938.

BÉCLÈRE, A. Le Cancer. Est-il une maladie virulente? *Presse Méd.*, 43, 737, 1935.

——— Le Cancer. Est-il une maladie virulente? II. Papillomes et cancer. *Presse Méd.*, 44, 337, 504, 1936.

BEIJERINCK, M. W. Ueber ein Contagium vivum fluidum als Ursache der Fleckenkrankheit der Tabaksblätter. *Centralbl. f. Bakteriol.*, Abt. II., 5, 27, 1899.

BORREL, A. Epithélioses infectieuses et Epithéliomas. *Ann. Inst. Pasteur*, 17, 81, 1903.

——— Le problème du cancer. *Bull. Inst. Pasteur.* 5, 497, 545, 593, 641, 1907.

CALMETTE, A., and GUÉRIN, C. Recherches sur la vaccine expérimentale. *Ann. Inst. Pasteur*, 15, 161, 1901.

CARREL, A. Le principe filtrant des sarcomes de la poule produits par l'arsenic. *Compt. rend. Soc. Biol.*, 93, 1083, 1925.

——— Un sarcome fusocellulaire produit par l'indol et transmissible par un agent filtrant. *Compt. rend. Soc. Biol.*, 93, 1278, 1925.

——— Essential Characteristics of a Malignant Cell. *J. American Med. Assn.*, 84, 157, 1925.

CIUFFO. Innesto positivo con filtrato di verruca vulgare. *Gior. ital. d. mal. ven.*, 42, 12, 1907.

CLAUDE, A. Properties of the Inhibitor Associated with the Active Agent of Chicken Tumor I. *American J. Cancer*, 37, 59, 1939.

——— and MURPHY, J. B. Transmissible Tumors of the Fowl. *Physiological Rev.*, 13, 246, 1933. (Bibliography.)

DAHMANN, H. Die Larynxpapillomatose. *Ztschr. f. Laryngol. u. Rhinol.*, 18, 383, 1929.

DAWSON, M. H., and SIA, R. H. P. In Vitro Transformation of Pneumococcal Types. I. A Technique for Inducing Transformation of Pneumococcal Types in Vitro. *J. Exper. Med.*, 54, 681, 1931.

DES LIGNERIS, M. J. A. Un cas de cancérisation *in vitro* par le dibenzanthracène. *Compt. rend. Soc. Biol.*, 120, 777, 1935.

DOLJANSKI, L., and TENENBAUM, E. Studies on Rous Sarcoma Cells Cultivated in Vitro. I. Cellular Composition of Pure Cultures of Rous Sarcoma Cells. *Cancer Research*, 2, 776, 1942.

DURAN-REYNALS, F. The Reciprocal Infection of Ducks and Chickens with Tumor-Inducing Viruses. *Cancer Research*, 2, 343, 1942.

——— The Infection of Turkeys and Guinea Fowls by the Rous Sarcoma Virus and the Accompanying Variations of the Virus. *Cancer Research*, 3, 569, 1943.

ELFORD, W. J. A New Series of Graded Collodion Membranes Suitable for General Bacteriological Use, Especially in Filterable Virus Studies. *J. Pathol. and Bacteriol.*, 34, 505, 1931.

ELLERMANN, V. Die übertragbare Hühnerleukose (Leukämie, Pseudoleukämie, Anämie, u.a.). Mit Beiträgen zur normalen Hämatologie der Hühner. Berlin, Springer, 1918.

ENGELBRETH-HOLM, J. Spontaneous and Experimental Leukemia in Animals. Edinburgh and London, Oliver & Boyd, 1942. (Bibliography.)

FOULDS, L. The Filterable Tumours of Fowls: A Critical Review. Eleventh Scientific Report, Imperial Cancer Research Fund. Supplement. London, Taylor & Francis, 1934. (Bibliography.)

FOULDS, L., and DMOCHOWSKI, L. Neutralizing and Complement-Fixing Properties of Antisera Produced by Fractionated Extracts of a Non-Filterable Dibenzanthracene Sarcoma. *British J. Exper. Pathol.*, 20, 458, 1939.

FUJINAMI, A., and INAMOTO, K., Ueber Geschwülste bei japanischen Haushühnern, insbesondere über einen transplantablen Tumor. *Ztschr. f. Krebsforsch.*, 14, 94, 1914.

FURTH, J. Lymphomatosis, Myelomatosis, and Endothelioma of Chickens Caused by a Filterable Agent. *J. Exper. Med.*, 58, 253, 1933.

GRATIA. Nature des ultravirus. In Levaditi and Lépine's Les Ultravirus des maladies humaines. Paris, Maloine, 1938.

GREEN, R. G., GOODLOW, R. J., EVANS, C. A., PEYTON, W. T., and TITRUD, L. A. Transmission of a Human Papilloma to Monkeys. *American J. Cancer*, 39, 161, 1940.

GRIFFITH, F. The Significance of Pneumococcal Types. *J. Hygiene*, 27, 113, 1928.

GYE, W. E. Tumours Transmissible with Viruses. Second Internat. Cancer Congress, Brussels, 1, 48, 1936.

——— and PURDY, W. J. The Cause of Cancer. London, Cassell, 1931.

HOLTFRETER, J. Kausalanalyse der Entwicklung. *Med. Welt*, 8, 633, 1934.

IWANOWSKI, D. Ueber die Mosaikkrankheit der Tabakspflanze. *Bull. Acad. Imp. Sci.*, St. Petersburg, 3, 67, 1892.

JÁRMAI, K. Tumorerzeugung mit dem Leukoseagens der Hühner. *Arch. Tierheilk.*, 69, 275, 1935. Cited by Engelbreth-Holm.

KIDD, J. G. The Masking Effect of Extravasated Antibody on the Rabbit Papilloma Virus (Shope). *J. Exper. Med.*, 70, 583, 1939.

——— A Distinctive Substance Associated with the Brown-Pearce Rabbit Carcinoma. I. Presence and Specificity of the Substance as Determined by Serum Reactions. *J. Exper. Med.*, 71, 335, 1940.

——— A Distinctive Substance Associated with the Brown-Pearce Rabbit Carcinoma. II. Properties of the Substance: Discussion. *J. Exper. Med.*, 71, 351, 1940.

——— and ROUS, P. Cancers Deriving from the Virus Papillomas of Wild Rabbits under Natural Conditions. *J. Exper. Med.*, 71, 469, 1940.

——— ——— A Transplantable Rabbit Carcinoma Originating in a Virus-Induced Papilloma and Containing the Virus in Masked or Altered Form. *J. Exper. Med.*, 71, 813, 1940.

KINGERY, L. B. The Etiology of Common Warts: Their Production in the Second Generation. *J. American Med. Assn.*, 76, 440, 1921. See also Wile and Kingery.

LEDINGHAM, J. C. G., and GYE, W. E. On the Nature of the Filtrable Tumour-Exciting Agent in Avian Sarcomata. *Lancet*, 1, 376, 1935.

LEVADITI, C., LÉPINE, P., et al. Les ultravirus des maladies humaines. Paris, Maloine, 1938.

LOEFFLER, F., and FROSCH. Summarischer Bericht über die Ergebnisse der Untersuchungen der Kommission zur Erforschung der Maul- und Klauenseuche bei dem Institut für Infektionskrankheiten in Berlin. *Centralbl. f. Bakteriol.*, Abt. I., 22, 257, 1897.

LUCKÉ, B. Carcinoma in Leopard Frog: Its Probable Causation by a Virus. *J. Exper. Med.*, 68, 457, 1938.

——— and SCHLUMBERGER, H. The Effect of Temperature on the Growth of Frog Carcinoma. I. Direct Microscopic Observations on Living Intraocular Transplants. *J. Exper. Med.*, 72, 321, 1940.

MCINTOSH, J. On the Nature of the Tumours Induced in Fowls by Injections of Tar. *British J. Exper. Pathol.*, 14, 422, 1933.

——— and SELBIE, F. R. Further Observations on Filterable Tumours Induced in Fowls by Injection of Tar. *British J. Exper. Pathol.*, 20, 49, 1939.

MELLANBY, E. Biochemical Studies on Cancer Growths. Eleventh Ann. Report, British Empire Cancer Campaign, 1934, p. 81.

MURPHY, J. B. Discussion of Some Properties of the Causative Agent of a Chicken Tumor. *Trans. Assn. American Physicians*, 46, 182, 1931.
——— and LANDSTEINER, K. Experimental Production and Transmission of Tar Sarcomas in Chickens. *J. Exper. Med.*, 41, 807, 1925.
NEUFELD, F., and LEVINTHAL, W. Beiträge zur Variabilität der Pneumokokken. *Ztschr. f. Immunitätsforsch.*, 55, 324, 1928.
NICOLLE, C. Naissance, vie et mort des maladies infectieuses. Paris, Alcan, 1930.
OBERLING, C., and GUÉRIN, M. Lesions tumorales en rapport avec la leucémie transmissible des poules. *Bull. Assn. française pour l'Etude du Cancer*, 22, 180, 1933.
——— ——— Nouvelles recherches sur la production de tumeurs malignes avec le virus de la leucémie transmissible des poules. *Bull. Assn. française pour l'Etude du Cancer*, 22, 326, 1933.
——— ——— La leucémie érythroblastique ou érythroblastose transmissible des poules. *Bull. Assn. Française pour l'Etude du Cancer*, 23, 38, 1934.
PEACOCK, P. R. Production of Tumours in the Fowl by Carcinogenic Agents: (1) Tar; (2) 1:2:5:6-Dibenzanthracene-Lard. *J. Pathol. and Bacteriol.*, 36, 141, 1933.
——— Studies of Fowl Tumours Induced by Carcinogenic Agents. II. Attempted Transmission by Cell-Free Material. *American J. Cancer*, 25, 49, 1935.
——— A Comparative Study of Filterable and Non-Filterable Fowl Tumours. Second Internat. Cong. for Microbiology, London, 1936, p. 97.
PENTIMALLI, F. Über die elektive Wirkung des Virus des Hühnersarkoms. *Ztschr. f. Krebsforsch.*, 22, 74, 1924.
——— Über Metastasenbildung beim Hühnersarkom. *Ztschr. f. Krebsforsch.*, 22, 62, 1925.
RAWLINS, T. E., and TAKAHASHI, W. N. The Nature of Viruses. *Science*, 87, 255, 1938.
RIVERS, T. M. Viruses and Virus Diseases. Stanford University Press, 1939.
——— and TILLETT, W. S. Further Observations on the Phenomena Encountered in Attempting to Transmit Varicella to Rabbits. *J. Exper. Med.*, 39, 777, 1924.
ROTHBARD, S., and HERMAN, J. R. Attempts to Propagate Fowl Tumors Produced by Benzpyrene and by Virus: Sites of Implantation Used: Eye of Chicken and Chorio-Allantoic Membrane of Chick Embryo. *Arch. Pathol.*, 28, 212, 1939.
ROUS, P. Transmission of a Malignant New Growth by Means of a Cell-Free Filtrate. *J. American Med. Assn.*, 56, 198, 1911.
——— The Virus Tumors and the Tumor Problem. *American J. Cancer*, 28, 233, 1936.
——— The Nearer Causes of Cancer. *J. American Med. Assn.*, 122, 573, 1943.
——— and BEARD, J. W. Progression to Carcinoma of Virus-Induced Rabbit Papillomas (Shope). *J. Exper. Med.*, 62, 523, 1935.
——— ——— Observations on Relation of Virus Causing Rabbit Papillomas to Cancers Deriving Therefrom: II. Evidence Provided by Tumors: General Considerations. *J. Exper. Med.*, 64, 401, 1936.
——— and KIDD, J. G. The Activating, Transforming, and Carcinogenic Effects of the Rabbit Papilloma Virus (Shope) upon Implanted Tar Tumors. *J. Exper. Med.*, 71, 787, 1940.
——— ——— Conditional Neoplasms and Subthreshold Neoplastic States: A Study of Tar Tumors of Rabbits. *J. Exper. Med.*, 73, 365, 1941. See also Kidd and Rous.
——— ——— and BEARD, J. W. Observations on Relation of Virus Causing Rabbit Papillomas to Cancers Deriving Therefrom: I. Influence of Host Species and of Pathogenic Activity and Concentration of Virus. *J. Exper. Med.*, 64, 385, 1936.
——— and LANGE, LINDA B. The Characters of a Third Transplantable Chicken Tumor Due to a Filterable Cause: A Sarcoma of Intracanalicular Pattern. *J. Exper. Med.*, 18, 651, 1913.
——— MURPHY, J. B., and TYTLER, W. H. Transplantable Tumors of the Fowl: A Neglected Material for Cancer Research. *J. American Med. Assn.*, 58, 1682, 1912.

Sanarelli, G. Das myxomatogene Virus. Beitrag zum Studium der Krankheitserreger ausserhalb des Sichtbaren. *Centralbl. f. Bakteriol.*, Abt. I., 23, 865, 1898.

Shope, R. E. A Transmissible Tumor-Like Condition in Rabbits. *J. Exper. Med.*, 56, 793, 1932.

——— A Filtrable Virus Causing a Tumor-Like Condition in Rabbits and Its Relationship to Virus Myxomatosum. *J. Exper. Med.*, 56, 803, 1932.

——— Infectious Papillomatosis of Rabbits. *J. Exper. Med.*, 58, 607, 1933.

——— Serial Transmission of Virus of Infectious Papillomatosis in Domestic Rabbits. *Proc. Soc. Exper. Biol. and Med.*, 32, 830, 1935. See also Andrewes and Shope.

Stanley, W. M. Chemical Studies on the Virus of Tobacco Mosaic. VI. The Isolation from Diseased Turkish Tobacco Plants of a Crystalline Protein Possessing the Properties of Tobacco-Mosaic Virus. *Phytopathol.*, 26, 305, 1936.

Storti, E., and Zaietta, A. Sui rapporti delle leucemia con le neoplasie sarcomatose: studio sulla patogenesi delle leucemia aviaria e tentativi di influenzamento del citotropismo del virus leucemico. *Arch. Sci. Med.*, 65, 897, 1938.

Sturm, E., and Murphy, J. B. Further Observations on an Experimentally Produced Sarcoma of the Chicken. *J. Exper. Med.*, 47, 493, 1928.

Syverton, J. T., and Berry, G. P. Carcinoma in the Cottontail Rabbit Following Spontaneous Virus Papilloma (Shope). *Proc. Soc. Exper. Biol. and Med.*, 33, 399, 1935.

Takahashi, W. N., and Rawlins, T. E. The Relation of Stream Double Refraction to Tobacco Mosaic Virus. *Science*, 81, 299, 1935.

——— ——— Stream Double Refraction of Preparations of Crystalline Tobacco-Mosaic Protein. *Science*, 85, 103, 1937. See also Rawlins and Takahashi.

Traub, E. A Filterable Virus Recovered from White Mice. *Science*, 81, 298, 1935.

——— The Epidemiology of Lymphocytic Choriomeningitis in White Mice. *J. Exper. Med.*, 64, 183, 1936.

Ullmann, E. V. On the Etiology of the Laryngeal Papilloma. *Acta Oto-Laryngologica*, 5, 317, 1923.

Waelsch, L. Erwiderung auf die Bemerkungen Cronquists zu meiner Arbeit: "Übertragungsversuche mit spitzem Kondylom." *Arch. f. Dermatol. u. Syph.*, 127, 909, 1919.

Webster, L. T. Inheritance of Resistance of Mice to Enteric Bacterial and Neurotropic Virus Infections. *J. Exper. Med.*, 65, 261, 1937.

White, A. W. M. A Study of Sarcoma of the Fowl Produced by Arsenic and Embryonic Pulp. *J. Cancer Research*, 11, 111, 1927.

Wile, U. J., and Kingery, L. B. The Etiology of Common Warts: Preliminary Report of an Experimental Study. *J. American Med. Assn.*, 73, 970, 1919. See also Kingery.

Woglom, W. H., and Warren, J. The Retention of Immunizing Power by the Shope Papilloma after Exposure to Ultraviolet Radiation. *American J. Cancer*, 37, 562, 1939.

V. CONCLUSION: ONE KIND OF CANCER OR MANY?

Andervont, H. B. The Influence of Foster Nursing upon the Incidence of Spontaneous Mammary Cancer in Resistant and Susceptible Mice. *J. National Cancer Institute*, 1, 147, 1940–41.

Andrewes, C. H., Ahlström, C. G., Foulds, L., and Gye, W. E. Reaction of Tarred Rabbits to the Infectious Fibroma Virus. *Lancet*, 2, 893, 1937.

Barnes, W. A., and Cole, R. K. The Effect of Nursing on the Incidence of Spontaneous Leukemia and Tumors in Mice. *Cancer Research*, 1, 99, 1941.

Bauer, K. H. Mutationstheorie der Geschwulstentstehung. Berlin, Springer, 1928.

Berry, G. P., and Dedrick, H. M. Method for Changing the Virus of Rabbit Fibroma (Shope) into That of Infections Myxomatosis (Sanarelli). *J. Bacteriol.*, 31, 50, 1936.

BITTNER, J. J. Relation of Nursing to the Extra-Chromosomal Theory of Breast Cancer in Mice. *American J. Cancer*, 35, 90, 1939.

——— Possible Method of Transmission of Susceptibility to Breast Cancer in Mice. *American J. Cancer*, 39, 104, 1940. (Bibliography.)

——— Changes in the Incidence of Mammary Carcinoma in Mice of the A Stock. *Cancer Research*, 1, 113, 1941.

BORREL, A. Parasitisme et Tumeurs. *Ann. Inst. Pasteur*, 24, 778, 1910.

BORST, M. Allgemeine Pathologie der maligne Geschwülste. Leipzig, Hirzel, 1924.

BOVERI, T. The Origin of Malignant Tumors. Baltimore, Williams & Wilkins Company, 1929. English translation by Marcella Boveri.

KALLMAN, F. J., and REISNER, D. Twin Studies on the Significance of Genetic Factors in Tuberculosis. *American Rev. Tuberculosis*, 47, 549, 1943.

KIDD, J. G., and ROUS, P. The Carcinogenic Effect of a Papilloma Virus on the Tarred Skin of Rabbits. II. Major Factors Determining the Phenomenon: The Manifold Effects of Tarring. *J. Exper. Med.*, 68, 529, 1938.

LACASSAGNE, A., and NYKA, W. Faible réaction, à l'injection intraveineuse du virus de Shope, au niveau des papillomes obtènus par badigeonnages au benzopyrène chez des lapins à hypophyse detruite. *Bull. Assn. française pour l'Etude du Cancer*, *26*, 154, 1937.

LEROUX, R., and SIMARD, L. C. Etude expérimentale du cancer du goudron chez le lapin. *Bull. et mémoires Soc. Anat.*, Paris, 95, 180, 1925.

LOCKHART-MUMMERY, J. P. The Origin of Cancer. London, Churchill, 1934.

LUDFORD, R. J. Chromosome Formation without Spindle Development in Cancer Cells, and Its Significance. Ninth Scientific Report, Imperial Cancer Research Fund. London, Taylor & Francis, 1930.

——— The Somatic Cell Mutation Theory of Cancer. Ninth Scientific Report, Imperial Cancer Research Fund. London, Taylor & Francis, 1930.

ROUS, P. The Virus Tumors and the Tumor Problem. *American J. Cancer*, 28, 233, 1936.

——— and KIDD, J. G. The Carcinogenic Effect of a Papilloma Virus on the Tarred Skin of Rabbits. Description of the Phenomenon. *J. Exper. Med.*, 67, 399, 1938.

——— ——— Activating, Transforming, and Carcinogenic Effects of Rabbit Papilloma Virus (Shope) on Implanted Tar Tumors. *J. Exper. Med.*, 71, 787, 1940. See also Kidd and Rous.

SHOPE, R. E. Complex Infections. *Arch. Pathol.*, 27, 913, 1939.

——— The Swine Lungworm as a Reservoir and Intermediate Host for Swine Influenza Virus. I. The Presence of Swine Influenza Virus in Healthy and Susceptible Pigs. *J. Exper. Med.*, 74, 41, 1941.

——— The Swine Lungworm as a Reservoir and Intermediate Host for Swine Influenza Virus. II. The Transmission of Swine Influenza Virus by the Swine Lungworm. *J. Exper. Med.*, 74, 49, 1941.

STRONG, L. C. Transplantation Studies on Tumors Arising Spontaneously in Heterozygous Individuals. I. Experimental Evidence for the Theory that the Tumor Cell Has Deviated from a Definitive Somatic Cell by a Process Analogous to Genetic Mutation. *J. Cancer Research*, 13, 103, 1929.

SUTTON, R. L., JR. Early Epidermal Neoplasia: Description and Interpretation. The Theory of Mutation in the Origin of Cancer. *Arch. Dermatol. and Syph.*, 37, 737, 1938.

WHITMAN, R. C. Somatic Mutations as a Factor in the Production of Cancer. A Critical Review of v. Hansemann's Theory of Anaplasia in the Light of Modern Knowledge of Genetics. *J. Cancer Research*, 4, 181, 1919.

——— A Study of Four Cases of Beginning Squamous-Cell Carcinoma of Cornifying Type. *J. Cancer Research*, 5, 155, 1920.

WOGLOM, W. H. Sarcoma 37 and the Virus Problem. *American J. Cancer*, 35, 374, 1939.

WOOD, F. C. Oral communication.

INDEX

ACARIDS, 67
Adaptation, 40, **44**
Adenocarcinoma, of frog kidney, 141
Adenoma, parasitic, of monkey's stomach, 73
Adenosarcoma, **28**, 33
Age, **5**, 24, 163
Ahlbohm, 85
Ahlström, 160
Alcohol, **19**, 87
Allen, 103, 104
Alloway, 134
Amines, aromatic, 105
Amino acids, effect on tumor growth, 53
o-Aminoazotoluene, 106
Andervont, 62, 100, 162
Ando, 106
Andrewes, 138, 160
Angioma, 11
Angiosarcoma, of fowl, filterable, 130
Aniline dyes, 105
Anissimova, 107
Anthracene, 95, 96, **97**
Antibodies, **56**, 133, 138, 145, 165
Antiseptics, resistance of viruses to, 132
Apolant, 39, 50
Appel, 55
Arsenous acid, 136
Aschoff, 55
Askanazy, 66
Asphalt, in carcinogenesis, 88
Assimilation, 129
Athrepsia, 47
Autonomy, **11**, 152; induced, 125, **129**, 157, 164, 169

BABCOCK, 107
Bacillus tumefaciens, 35
Bacteriophage, 111, **117**, 118, 123, 164
Bang, 64
Bard, 14, 139
Bashford, 39, 50, 51
Basset, 126
Bauer, 167
Baumann, 63, 106
Beard, 63
Beauty spots, 26
Becquerel, 61
Beijerinck, 111
Benzanthracene, 97
Benzene nucleus, 96
Benzpyrene, 25, **96**, 98, 100, 159
Berenblum, 109
Berger, 6
Berry, 146, 156
Besredka, 55, 56
Betanaphthylamine, 105
Bibliography, 170
Bichat, 12, 13
Biette, 38
Bile, 17, **102**, 104, 109, 151
Bilharziasis, in etiology, 66
Billroth, 18
Biltris, 61
Biotropism, 115
Birefringence of flow, 121
Bischoff, 54
Bittner, 82, 162
Blastema, 14
Blatta americana, 69
Blatta orientalis, 69
Bloch, 61, 95, 109
Blum, 63
Boggess, 63
Bonne, 48, 71, 73, 74
Bonser, 103, 105
Borrel, 36, 39, 67, 68, 70, 71, 72, 73, 75, 112, 116, 129, 148, 157, 158, 161
Borst, 152
Boveri, 23, 65, 167
Bridgework, 20
Brothers, cancer in, 83
Broussais, 18
Browning, 107
Brumpt, 71
Brunschwig, 72
Bullock, 73, 75
Burns, malignant change in, 19, **64**, 153; X ray, 59
Burrows, 103
Butter, effect on tumor growth, 53
Butter yellow, 106

CALMETTE, 117
Cancer. *See also* Carcinoma
Cancer, aniline dye, 19, **105**; betel nut, 19; campaigns, **6**, 16; cause of, *see* Etiology; a cellular disorder, 8, **17**; centers, 7; chimney sweep's, 19, **88**; a conditioned disorder, 153; cotton spinner's, 19, **88**; *à deux*, 36; districts, 35; earliest reference to, 10; embryonal ori-

Cancer (*continued*)
gin of, 26; experimental, 38; families, **83**, 86; frequency of, 2; growth capacity of, 22; industrial, 19, **88**, 102, 105; interest in, 1; Kangri (in Kashmir), 19; knowledge of, 10; nature of, 1, **10**, 27, 31, 44; one kind or many? 150; "rejuvenation" of, 5; Schneeberg, 19; social importance of, 2; spiroptera, 69; spontaneous, **44**, 58; strains, 77; tar, 19, 25, 31, **89**, 159; transplantable, **44**, 58, 165; in twins, 29, 30, **83**, 87; X-ray, 19, 25, **59**, 60, 63, 64, 65
"Cancer cages," **36**, 84
Cancer cell, defensive reactions against, 48; dormant, 45; specific nutrient for, 47
"Cancer houses," 35, **36**, 84
Cancerophobia, **1**, 7
"Cancers in the cradle," 166
Carbohydrates, effect on tumor growth, 53
Carcinogenesis, **87**, 109; susceptibility of various species, **99**, 109
Carcinogenic compounds, 80, **87**, 94, 103, 105, 106, 107, 108, 109, 151, 153, 154, 157, 159; hydrocarbons, **94**, 110
Carcinogenic viruses, 67, 70, 75, **129**
Carcinoma. *See also* Cancer
Carcinoma, 14; basal cell, in rat, 99; gastric, in rat, 67; mammary, in mouse, 79, **81**, 100, 103, 158, 162, in rat, 103
Carcinos, 10
Carcinosis, **46**, 49
Carrel, 42, 53, 132, 136
Castration, **103**, 108
Catalysts, 123
Cause. *See* Etiology
Cazin, 90
Cell, cancer, differentiation of, 22; embryonal, 26, differentiation of, 30, growth capacity of, 27, resemblance to cancer cell, 31; multiplication of, 13; specificity, 14; theory, 12; tumor, growth capacity of, **27**, 49
Champy, 107
Chance, hypothesis of, 23
Change, malignant, **21**, 23, 31, 32, 33, 137, 168, 169; precancerous, 20, **21**; sarcomatous, 43, **50**
Character, cancer, **81**, 85
Cholanthrene, 101
Cholesterol, 53, **102**
Chondroma, 11, **28**, 32
Chondrosarcoma, 33
Chordoma, 28
Chromosomes, 65, **78**, 167, 169
Ciuffo, 147
Claude, 132, 134, 138
Clemmesen, 72
Cloudman, 82
Clunet, 46, 61
"Coccidia," 35
Cohnheim, 26, 30, 32
Cold sore, 117
Collard, 12
Collip, 104
Compte, 13
Condyloma, 148
Connective tissue, **14**, 21, 24, 32, 132
Contagion, **35**, 163
Contamin, 50
Cook, 96, 103, 110
Cornil, 38
Costa, 53
Cramer, 51, 72, 104
Cropper, 94, 96
Croton oil, 109
Cultivation, in vitro, 32, **42**, 48, 49, 100, 132, 137
Cure, spontaneous, 165
Curie, 61
Curtis, 73, 75, 157
Cysticercus fasciolaris, 67, **73**
Cytoplasm, effect of X rays on, 66
Cytotoxic sera, 57
Cytotropism, **115**, 141

DAELS, 61
Dahmann, 148
Darier, 35
Dawson, 134
Death certificates, unreliability of, 3
Dedrick, 156
Deelman, 95
de Martel, 38, 56
Demodex folliculorum, 67
Dentures, 20
Descartes, 13, 17
des Ligneris, 21, 110, 137
Deslongchamps, 69, 70
Diagnosis, 2, 3, **4**, 7, 15
Diathesis, 93
Dibenzanthracene, **97**, 99, 100, 101
Diet, in carcinogenesis, 19, **71**, 106; in treatment, 52
Differentiation of cancer cell, 22; embryo, 30; in etiology, 22
di Mario, 4
p-Dimethylaminoazobenzene, 106
Distoma hepaticum, 74
Dmochowski, 137

Dobrovolskaïa-Zavadskaïa, 80
Dodds, 103
Doljanski, 132
Dominance, **77**, 80, 81
Doyen, 34
Dreyfuss, 95
Drosophila eggs, effect of X rays on, 65
Duffield, 4
Dumas, 12
Dunning, 73, 75
Durand, 38
Duran-Reynals, 137, 141, 155
Durante, 26

EARTHWORM, as virus carrier, 158
Ehrlich, 39, 47, 48, 49, 50, 56, 58, 75
Elford, 114
Ellermann, 139
Emboli, 45
Embryo, chick, transplantation into, 42
Embryoma, 29
Embryonal, *see also* Cell; rests, 26; tissues, in sarcomatogenesis, 136
Endocrine glands, in treatment, 54; tumors of, 15
Endothelioma, filterable, of fowl, 130
Engelbreth-Holm, 100, 141
Enzymes, **123**, 129, 135
Epithelioma, 14
Epithelium, **14**, 21, 24
Estrus, 103
Etiology, 11, 14, 16, 18, 25, 33, **59**, 66, 75, 87, 94, 150, 157, 159, 160; multiple, 86, **152**, 167
Evans, 148
Excision. *See* Surgery
Experimental method, limitations of, 52
Extirpation, and metastasis, 46
Eye, transplantation into, 41, **42**

FACTORS, extrachromosomal, 82, **161**; hereditary, **75**, 80, 83, 94, 100, 104, 156; multiple, 82
Falin, 107
Falko, 71
Fasciola hepatica, 74
Favre, 116
Fayet, 38
Feinberg, 35
Ferments, 123
Feygin, 60
Fibiger, 67, 69, 70, 71, 158
Fibroadenoma, mammary, of rat, 44
Fibroblast, susceptibility to virus, 132
Fibroma, **11**, 28; virus, in rabbit, **143**, 156
Fielding, 71
Fieser, 98
Findlay, 63
Fischer, Bernhard, 106
Fischer-Wasels, 93, 106
Flory, 94
Fluorescence, 96
Folliculin, **102**, 103, 104
Food. *See also* Diet
Food, hot, in etiology, 19
Foreign bodies, 20
Foulds, 62, 137, 160
Fridericia, 72
Frieben, 60
Frog, adenocarcinoma in, 141
Frosch, 111
Fujimaki, 71
Fujinami, 130, 138
Fujiwara, 106
Furth, 99, 141

GALEB, 68
Galen, 10, 11, 12, 17, 167
Gall-stones, 19
Gametes, in heredity, 76
Gardner, 103, 104
Generation, spontaneous, 118, **127**
Genes, **65**, 167
Genetics. *See also* Heredity
Genetics, **75**, 160
Genital tract, tumors of, 24, **104**
Geschickter, 103
Glioma, **33**, 83
Gluge, 13
Gongylonema neoplasticum, **69**, 157
Goodlow, 148
Grady, 63
Gratia, 119, 127
Green, 148
Greene, 42, 80
Griffith, 134
Gromzeva, 107
Gudjonsson, 72
Guérin, 56, 62, 110, 117, 140
Guinea pig, refractory to tar cancer, 91
Gulbransen, 107
Gye, 133, 160

HAALAND, 39, 50
Haga, 90
Hahn, 38
Hallion, 17
Hanau, 38, 39, 90
Harrison, 42
Heidenhain, 43
Henshaw, 65

Hellner, 62
Hepaticola gastrica, 74
Heredity, 2, 14, 39, **75**, 83, 100, 150, 157, 160; extrachromosomal, 82, **161**; in man, 83; mendelian, 161
Héricourt, 57
Herlitz, 63
Herman, 137
Herpes, **117**, 162
Heterozygosity, 77
Hieger, 96, 97, 110
Hippocrates, 1, 10
Histology, **12**, 16
Histosporidium carcinomatosum, 35
Holtfreter, 134
Holtz, 63
Homozygosity, 77
Hooke, 12
Hormones, 11, 81, 85, **102**, 151, 156
Horning, 104
Hueper, 105
Huldschinsky, 63
Hybridization, 76; test, 84
Hybrids, **77**, 80, 82
Hydrochloric acid, sarcoma induced with, 107
Hyperplasia, **10**, 22, 25
"Hypnosis of positive cases," **22**, 36
Hypothesis, athreptic, 47; embryonal, 18, **26**, 59; hereditary, *see* Heredity; humoral, 17; irritation, **18**, 30, 32, 59, 70, 92, 107, 109; lymphatic, **13**, 17; microbic, 33; mutagen, 135; virus, **129**, 154, 157, 159, 160

IMMUNITY, 39, **51**, 55, 75, 133, 143; *see also* Panimmunity
Inamoto, 130
Inclusion bodies, 120, **141**
Indol, 136
Industrial cancer, **88**, 94, 102, 105
Infection versus neoplasia, **33**, 38, 41
Inflammation. *See* Irritation, chronic
Inheritance. *See* Heredity
Injury, in etiology, 79, **81**, 87
In vitro. *See* Cultivation in vitro
Irritation, chronic, **18**, 31, 32, 94, 108
Isoprene tar, 95
Itchikawa, 89

JÁRMAI, 141
Jensen, 39
Jonkhoff, 61
Jundell, 63

KALLMAN, 161
Kennaway, 95, 110
Kidd, 108, 144, 145, 156, 159, 164
Kingery, 147
Kinosita, 106
Kirby-Smith, 63
Kleinenberg, 109, 110
Knox, 71
Koch, 152
Korteweg, 161

LACASSAGNE, 61, 103, 104, 159
Laënnec, 14, 15
Landsteiner, 137
Lange, 130
Larrimore, 72
Latent period, 90, **101**, 105, 106, 131, 149, 154, 159, 168
Lathrop, 77
Lavedan, 108
Lawson, 103
Lebert, 13
Lecithin, 53
Leese, 71
Leeuwenhoek, 12
Lefèvre, 100
Le Noble, 38
Leroux, 159
Leukemia, 99, 100, **139**, 148, 159, 162
Leukoplakia, 19
Levinthal, 134
Lewin, 50
Leyden, 14
Leydig, 13
Lipids, 53
Lipoma, **11**, 28
Little, 80, 82, 161
Liver, cancer of, induced, 106
Lobstein, 26
Localization, factor for, 82
Lockhart-Mummery, 167
Loeb, Leo, 39, 50, 77, 81, 103, 107
Loeffler, 111
Long, 54
Lorenz, 99
Lucké, 141
Ludford, 167, 169
Lüdin, 61
Lumière, 24, 36
Lumsden, 48, 57
Lung, carcinoma of, in mice, 100
Lynch, 80, 81, 161

MACDOWELL, 80, 161
Macheboef, 126
Macrophage, susceptibility to virus, 132

Maisin, 93, 95
Malformations, 32
Malignancy, factor for, 82
"Malignant mutation," 169
Marsh, 81
Martland, 62
Masson, 11
Masugi, 57
Mayneord, 96, 97
McCoy, 68, 106
McFarland, 83
McIntosh, 136, 137
Meade, 83
Meat, effect on tumor growth, 53
Mellanby, 137
Membranulae, 12
Mendel, 76
Mendelian laws, **76**, 80, 82
Ménétrier, 22
Meningoencephalic gliosis, 33
Mesothorium, 62
Metals, effect on tumor growth, 55
Metastases, 15, 39, 44, **46**, 47, 49, 70, 131, 140, 144, 145; red, 131
Methylcholanthrene, 17, **98**, 99, 101, 102, 109
Mice, cancer and noncancer strains, **75**, 77, 80, 161; inbred strains, 44, **78**; leukemia in, 99, 100
Michalowsky, 107
Microbes, **33**, 110, 112, 118, 128, 155, 161, 164, 165, 166
Micron, 110
Microscope, 12, **16**, 20; electron, 113
"Milk influence," 82, **162**
Miller, 106
Millimicron, 111
Millimu, 111
Miner, 106
Mites, 67
Mitosis, 21, **23**, 65, 100, 117, 118, 125, 168
Mole, **26**, 28, 30, 32
Monkey, tumors of stomach in, 73
Monsters, 29
Moreau, 38, 39
Mori, 106
Mosaic diseases, 111
Mother's mark, 26
Müller, J., 13, 26
Muller, 65
Multiplication by induction, 125, **129**
Murphy, 42, 92, 100, 130, 134, 135, 137
Murray, J. A., 39, 51, 77
Murray, W. S., 82
Muspicea borreli, 158
Mutation, **23**, 65, 157, 167
Myxoma, infectious, of rabbit, **142**, 156
Myxosarcoma, filterable, of fowl, 130

NAGAYO, 42
Nakahara, 106
Naudin, 76
Nematode worms, **68**, 74, 158
Neoplasia versus infection, **33**, 38, 41
Neufach, 109, 110
Neufeld, 134
Neuroepithelioma, **28**, 33
Neurofibromatosis. *See* Recklinghausen's disease
Neurosarcoma, 33
Neurospongioma, 33
Nevus. *See* Mole
Nicolas, 116
Nicolle, 8, 128
Nishimura, 71
Niven, 107
Nochtia nochti, 74
Nonaka, 107
Notochord, 28
Nucleus, **23**, 65, 66, 168; benzene, 96
Nyka, 159

OBERLING, 6, 33, 62, 93, 140
Oil, fuel, 88; lubricating, 88; olive, 53
Okada, 106
Omnis cellula e cellula, 13
Onchocerca volvulus, 74
Opisthorchis felineus, 66
Organizers, 133
Osteoma, 11
Osteosarcoma, 62, **130**
Ovaries, 81, **103**
Overholser, 104
Ovum, 18

PAGET, 26
Panimmunity, 56
Papilloma, in man, 105, **147**; in rabbit, 143, carcinomatous change, 144; in rat, 70, **72**; Shope, **143**, 166, 168; tar, **89**, 108; transmissibility in man, 147
Pappenheimer, 72
Paramecium, 101
Parasites, **66**, 151, 153, 157, 162, 169
Parasitism, obligate intracellular, 116, **128**, 155
Passey, 71, 158
Pasteur, 33, 111, 129
Paulsen, 83
Peacock, 132, 136, 164

Pentimalli, 132
Perlmann, 105
Permeability, cell membrane, 66
Pessaries, 20
Petroleum, 88
Peyrilhe, 38
Peyton, 148
Phenylalanine, 53
Pierson, 104
Pitch, 88
Plants, tumors of, 35
Plummer-Vinson syndrome, 85
Polyp, 83
Populations, aging of, 5
Port-wine stain, 28
Pott, 88, 89
Proenzyme, 124
Proferment, 124
Proteins, 53
Proteoses, 49
Protozoa, 35
Provirus, 124
Putnoky, 42
Putschar, 63

RABBIT, fibroma, 143; myxoma, 142; papilloma, 143; tar cancer, 25, **89**
Radiation, resistance of viruses, to, 164
Radioactivity, 25, **63**
Radiodermatitis, **59**, 61
Radiotherapy, **7**, 15, 45, 56
Radium, in causation, 61, **62**; in sarcomatogenesis, 19, **61**
Raileanu, 93
Rappin, 33
Rasmussen, 72
Raspail, 12
Rat, carcinoma in, basal cell, 99; mammary, 103
Rawlins, 121
Rays, carcinogenic, 59; heat, in etiology, 63, **64**; infrared, in etiology, **63**, 64; light, **63**, 64; ultraviolet, in etiology, 63, in carcinogenesis, **63**, 102, 109, in microscopy, 112
Récamier, 26
Recessiveness, **77**, 80, 81, 82, 84
Recklinghausen's disease, 28, **29**, 83
Recurrence, **33**, 46
Reding, 93
Regeneration, 22
Rehn, 105
Reisner, 161
Remak, 26
Revelatory conditions, **81**, 86, 100
Rhabdomyoma, **28**, 33
Rhoads, 106
Ribbert, 32
Richet, 57
Richter, 80, 161
Ringworm, 163
Rivers, 120
Robson, 103
Roentgen, 59
Roentgen cancer. *See* Cancer, X-ray
Roessle, 57
Roffo, 63, 64, 94, 102
Ross, 94, 96
Rothbard, 137
Rous, 25, 108, 130, 131, 134, 144, 145, 146, 155, 156, 159, 164
Roussy, 46, 62
Roux, 111
Ruffer, 66
Rusch, 63, 106
Russell, 50

SABIN, 63
Sailor's skin, 18
Sanarelli, 142, 143
Sandground, 73, 74
Sannié, 109
Saphir, 55
Sarcoma, 14; filterable, of fowl, 130; induced, with carcinogenic hydrocarbons, 99, **101**, with follicular hormone, 104, with hydrochloric acid, 107, by injury, **79**, 81, with liver extracts, 109, with sugar, 107; radium, 61; rat's liver, 67, **73**; relation to leukemia, 141; styryl 430, 107; tar, **91**, 136; tomato, 34
Sasaki, 106
Sawtschenko, 35
Scarlet R, 105
Scars, malignant change in, **24**, 64
Schabad, 92, 100, 109, 110
Schär, 105
Scheurlen, 34
Schistosoma japonicum, 74
Schistosoma mansoni, 74
Schistosomum haematobium, 66
Schleiden, 12
Schlumberger, 141
Schürch, 61, 63, 94
Schwann, 12
Segregation, 77
Selection, **22**, 23
Selenium, 55
Selye, 104
Seurat, 71
Sex, in causation, 5, 24, **81**, 103; cells, effect of X rays on, 65

Shear, 101, 106
Shimkin, 62
Shingles, 162. *See also* Herpes
Shope, 143, 144, 147, 156, 158
Sia, 134
Simard, 159
Sisters, cancer in, 83
Slosse, 93
Slye, 78, 81, 83
Smith, E. F., 35
Smith, G. M., 103
Sobotka, 109
Somatic cells, effect of X rays on, 65
Soot, 20, **88**
Spemann, 133
Spirochetes, 35
Spiroptera neoplastica, 69
Spores, 164
Staehler, 105
Stanley, 121, 122
Statistics, **2**, 36, 83, 84
Steiner, 110
Sterols, **102**, 104
Stewart, 99
Storti, 141
Stroma, defined, 50; sarcomatous change in, 43, **50**
Strong, L. C., 80, 103, 167
Strong, R. P., 74
Strongylus filaria, 74
Sturm, 92, 100, 137
Styryl 430, 107
Sugar, effect on tumor growth, 53
Sugiura, 106
Sunlight, in carcinogenesis, 102; in etiology, 20, 33, **63**, 85
Suntzeff, 107
Surgery, 7, **21**, 45, 46
Sutton, 167
Swine influenza, 158
Syphilis, **19**, 148
Syverton, 146

TAENIA crassicollis, 67, **73**
Takahashi, 121
Takizawa, 107
Tar, absorbed, 93; active agent in, **94**, 102; carcinoma, 31, **89**, 159, 163; fractionation of, 94; fractions, ultraviolet fluorescence spectrum, 96; lesions, 92; remote tumors produced with, 92; sarcoma, 91, **136**; susceptibility of various species, 88, **91**, 109
Tarring, technic of, 90
Tenenbaum, 132
Teratology, 29
Teratoma, **29**, 31
Testis, induced tumors of, 107
Testosterone, 103
Thomson, 104
Thorium, **62**, 66
Thorotrast, **62**, 64
Thyroid, carcinoma of, in mice, **82**, 84
Tissue culture. *See* Cultivation in vitro
Tissues, susceptibility to carcinogenesis, **91**, 99, to X-rays, 100; tumors induced with, 136
Titrud, 148
Tobacco, 19, 87, **94**
Transformation. *See* Change, malignant
Transplantation, adaptation to, 43; autologous, **38**, 56; heterologous, 38, **40**, 42, 43, 47, 48, 138, 141, 144; homologous, **38**, 40, 141; technic, 41; tumors, 38; zig-zag, 47
Traub, 120
Trauma. *See* Injury
Treatment, in animals, 53, **55**; in man, **7**, 15, 21, 45, 52, 56, 65, 100
Trephones, 46
Truhaut, 109
Tryptophan, 53
Tsutsui, 90
Tubangui, 71
Tumor, the induced, 59; spontaneous, 40, 56, **58**; transplantable, 38, **40**
Tumors, benign, 11, transplantable, 44; classification of, 4, **10**, 14; concordant, 87; congenital, 26, 33; discordant, 87; dysembryoplastic, 28; embryonal, **26**, 167; filterable, 41, **130**; function by, 15; hyperplastic, 11; remote, **92**, 99, 132; structure of, 14, **16**; true, **11**, 32; virus, 129, in birds, 130, frogs, 141, mammals, **142**, 168, man, 147, natural transmission of, 159
Turpentine, 109
Twins, **29**, 83, 87, 161
Tyrosine, 53
Tytler, 130
Tyzzer, 77

U*EHLINGER*, 61, 63
Ulcer, gastric, relation to cancer, 19
Ullmann, 147
Ultracentrifugation, 139
Ultraviolet rays, 63, 96, 102, 109, **112**; fluorescence spectrum, 96
Unna, 18
Uranium, 61

VECTORS, 158
Vesiculae, 12
Vimtrup, 72
Vinzent, 61
Virchow, 13, 14, 15, 20, 66
Virus III, **120**, 121
Virus diseases, dissemination of, 158; susceptibility to, 161
Virus tumors, 129
Viruses, autonomy of, 126; carcinogenic, 110, stability of, 165, ubiquity of, 163; cultivation of, **115**, 125; cytolytic, **118**, 125; cytostimulant, 125; cytotropic, **115**, 132; ectodermotropic, 116; endogenous and exogenous, 135; filtration of, 111, **114**; free, **145**, 155, 164; general nature of, **111**, 128; inapparent, *see* latent; latent, **118**, 137; masked, **145**, 155, 158, 164; mesenchymotropic, 116; multiplication by induction, 125, **129**, 157; multiplicity, **155**, 166; mutation, **141**, 155; neuroepidermal, 116; neurotropic, 116; origin of, 128; particle size, **112**, 126; purification, **121**, 133; rapidity of action, 148; resistance to various agents, 126, 131, **132**, 141, 158, 164; selectivity, **115**, 140, 141, 144, 148; staining, 112; tumors, 129; ubiquity, **126**, 154; ultracentrifugation, 115
Vital induction, 125, **129**, 157, 164, 169
Vitamins, 52, **53**, 71, 102, 107
Voegtlin, 53
von Hamm, 63
von Wassermann, 55

WAALER, 84
Waelsch, 148
Wahlgren, 63
Warren, 123
Wart. *See also* Papilloma
Wart, venereal, 148
Warthin, 82, 84
Wassink, 84, 85
Wave length, 112
Webster, 115
Wells, H. Gideon, 33, 78
White, 136
Whitman, 167
Wile, 147
Wiley, 105
Winterstein, 94
Woglom, 39, 123, 160
Wolfe, 105
Wollman, 126
Wood, F. C., 164

X RAYS, 4, 15, 19, 25, 55, **59**, 63, 64, 65, 75, 80, 89, 91, 94, 100, 108, 132, 152, 156, 164, 167
Xeroderma pigmentosum, **33**, 60, 63, 85, 104

YAMAGIWA, 89
Yokogawa, 71
Yoshida, 106

ZAIETTA, 141
Zinc salts, 107
Zymogen, 124